I HAVE CANCER BUT IT DOESN'T HAVE ME

LLOYD DEITSCH

authorHOUSE®

AuthorHouse™
1663 Liberty Drive
Bloomington, IN 47403
www.authorhouse.com
Phone: 1-800-839-8640

Published by AuthorHouse   04/24/2012

ISBN: 978-1-4685-6234-7 (sc)
ISBN: 978-1-4685-6233-0 (e)

Library of Congress Control Number: 2012904700

HAPPY NEW YEAR
2008

I WOULD LIKE TO DEDICATE THIS BOOK
TO MY MOTHER WHO DIED OF COLON
CANCER IN THE YEAR OF 1973 AT THE
AGE OF FIFTY-SEVEN

MAY GOD GRANT YOU HEALTH FOR MANY YEARS

THIS IS MY STORY

My story really begins early in the fall of the year of 2003. I was starting to experience the loss of some of my strength. My left arm and leg to be exact. No real ache or pain.

I had over extended the bottom of my left foot a couple of months ago. I was transferring a patient from his bed to his wheel chair at my work site. I was working as a medical assistant at a health care site. I was taken by fellow worker to a company doctor. He put me in a boot to support my weight, keeping off my foot. I missed a couple of weeks work. First work I had missed in three years. The foot seemed improved after a time.

A short time later, my knee on both of my lets started giving me a whole lot of trouble. I was now having pain in both my legs and both of my knees. I began to think that maybe it was actually caused by the weather. The weather was starting to cool down. Fall and winter were approaching.

I was beginning to slow down on my job. I was employed by Great Bend Health and Rehabilitation. The job of medical assistant requires that you are in good health. My leg and arm had gotten so bad I just couldn't do my job as it should be done.

I finally decided to check into my possibility to draw Social Security. I called the Social Security Office in Hutchinson Kansas for my retirement wage information. After several days of talking on the telephone and filling out a lot of papers for the Social Security Office, I had now made my decision to retire. It took a lot of careful thought and consideration by me and my family. On the 17th of November, 2003, it was official, after I signed my name on some official looking papers. I was now a member of the Over-the-Hill Gang. I was now retired. Not wanting to lose my job and being without any income I retired. No more of that normal 2:00-10:00 P.M. rat race.

Winter was now rapidly bursting on the scene and the cold weather was making my knees and legs hurt even worse. I had no idea what was going on. It was starting to worry me, you know not being able to walk very well or very far.

About this time my daughter decided that she needed to take care of us, mother and dad. Her mother has already had 3 heart attacks. So

1

she went out and bought a big house in the city of Hoisington, Kansas. Just one city block from Main Street. The house used to be a duplex, which worked very nicely for us. She moved us right into her newly boughten home. Her and our granddaughter live in one end and her mother and I live in the other end of the house.

But not all things, as I think back, were really that bad. I remember one day I had a (M.R.I.) and the table I was on was higher than the (M.R.I.) table. There wasn't any trouble at all getting down on the (M.R.I.) table, but when I needed to go back up on the other table, it took 6 people to put me back up on my table. The difference was at least 10 inches or more, but we made it.

Now back to my story. I was starting to have some major problems getting around. I had been doctoring for sometime with my family doctor, Dr. Lee in Great Bend, Kansas. He had started testing me. After many many tests and blood work he was thinking my problems were some form of arthritis or maybe a muscle degeneration of some kind.

I am now doing a lot of blood testing and bone scans at (C.K.M.C.) Center Kansas Medical Center in Great Bend, Kansas. We continue to doctor for what we are calling a form of arthritis, but nothing seems to be working out for me. I visit my doctor regularly looking for any kind of new and positive answers.

I am now losing control of my left side, my arm, hand and my leg down to my feet. It is getting harder and harder to hold a cup full of coffee, a fork or even a spoon. That makes it real hard to eat. You drop a lot of your food and drink.

I am doing a lot of blood testing at (C.K.M.C.) in Great Bend. But I am still coming up empty. Time is passing very rapidly or it seemed to me like many months have gone by since I started having these balance and control problems.

I have had x-rays, M.R.I., CTS, Pet Scans and Bone Scan and no luck. I also have blood test (C.B.C. C.M.P. B.M.P. TSH) and many, many more blood tests. I remember on one afternoon I had a total of 27 x-rays in the Hospital in Great Bend (C.K.M.C.) but things are still coming up as always, no new answer or conclusions.

The weather is now starting to change as spring is about to burst on the scene, but we still don't have any new answers and I am not getting even worse. As spring comes with the warm weather I am hoping warm weather makes me feel better.

Dr. Lee, my family doctor has decided to sent me to a Urologist to have my prostate checked out. The Urologist, Dr. Witt, in Hoisington, Kansas, then checked out my prostate. My blood test shows my (P.S.A.) was at 2100, WOW. He scheduled me for a complete slate of prostate biopsies. My (P.S.A.) is getting higher all the time. We had another blood test. My (P.S.A.) is now at (2500) and it should be at (4.4) or a little less.

One week later I had a total of 8 biopsies that were taken at Dr. Witt's Office in Hoisington, Kansas on August 5, 2004. It was very warm as summer was having its last fling before the seasons started to change. I was now facing a very real possibility of having prostate cancer. This was real scary to me in the beginning, but how could losing control of your left side have to do with your prostate?

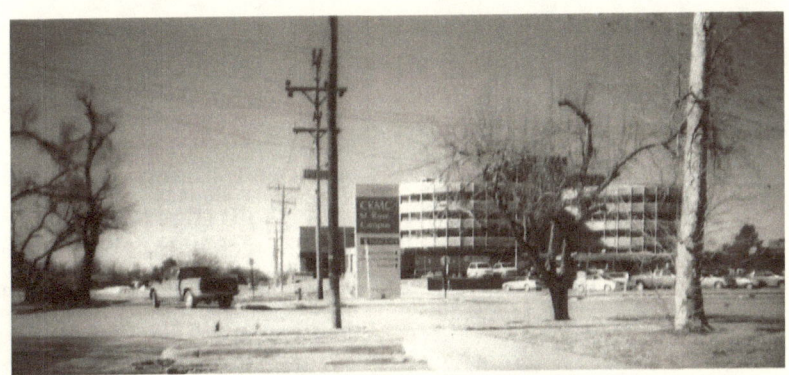

Great Bend Hospital

The biopsies are taken by inserting a tube up the rectum. Inside of this tube a wire is inserted which will be used to operate a tiny floodlight, a pair of mini clippers and a very small camera.

The clippers are used to take very small samples of prostate tissue (skin) from different spots on the prostate. The camera and light helps light the prostate so the camera can project pictures onto a small TV screen. They are then sent to the laboratory in Oklahoma for a reading to determine if there are any abnormal or cancerous cells.

I had a total of 8 biopsies that were taken and they all came back normal, no cancer cells. This was a big relief for me, but now we are again back where we started again except, my (P.S.A.) is high and getting higher all the time.

My (P.S.A.) was continuing to climb. It had now gone up to a whopping 2700. All my strength is now gone. I had to be helped in and out of my bed. I also have to be put in a wheelchair. I can't go to the restroom without the assistance of a lot of help. I just can't walk anymore at all or do much of anything else.

The last time I went to see Dr. Lee before I went to the hospital (C.K.M.C.), he came out of the car to examine me. It took three people to put me in my car when they were taking me to the Great Bend Hospital. It was almost impossible to get me into the car at home and out of the car at the hospital (C.K.M.C.) in Great Bend, Kansas to a wheelchair.

I was completely paralyzed on my left side. I still don't know what is wrong with me. I can't move my left arm, my leg or my hand. I am not really wheelchair bound, because I can't walk at all.

I have now come to a place, or a time in my life when I begin thinking I am on my way out or about to leave this life as we know it. I just knew my days were numbered or I was about to cash my last check.

They put me in the hospital in Great Bend, Kansas (C.K.M.C.). Dr. Lee told me, when he put me in the hospital, he was calling in a cancer specialist by the name of Dr. Fesen from the Heartland Cancer Center in Great Bend, Kansas. Dr. Fesen is well respected among doctors throughout the United States for his work in the cancer field.

Dr. Lee feels, or is almost sure that I had some form of cancerous or abnormal cells somewhere in my system, with my high P.S.A., but where that is, is the big question. Yet to be answered with more tests and more scans & M.R.I.

I was getting myself settled in at the hospital (C.K.M.C.) if in fact you can settle yourself in when you are in a wheelchair. I had to wait to see just what would be happening next. I didn't have to wait very long though. Guess what! More blood tests, scans, and M.R.I. I had breakfast and dinner in between tests. I got a goodnights sleep and woke up early the next morning. I was greeted by a new visitor, Dr. Fesen and his (P.A.) physicians assistant. Breakfast would have to wait for a little while now.

The first thing I heard from Dr. Fesen, when he came in, was "why did I leave this go on for so long?" I tried to explain to him about my dad having neck and back surgery and my brother Don having neck surgery. Dr. Fesen informed me that we didn't need Dr. Dad or Dr. Don because he was now on the case.

He then proceeded to inform me that we were going to a much bigger hospital in the city of Hutchinson, Kansas. I asked him why? I was already in a hospital now and it was close to my home.

Dr. Fesen told me they had better trained staff in this field. They also have a lot more and better medical equipment. I can't hardly fight this move under these conditions. His staff was a lot better trained to work cancer patients than they were here. At the Great Bend Hospital hear near my home. So this discussion was settled very quickly.

I was now on my way to a hospital in Hutchinson, Kansas, by way of the Hoisington Ambulance Service. My daughter made the arrangements, because she is employed part time by the Hoisington Ambulance Service in my hometown.

The ambulance driver, whom I know personally, told me he would only be hitting half of the holes on the way down to Hutchinson and the other half of the holes on the way back to Hoisington.

When I arrived I was being checked in, getting all my paper work done and being put in a room, when I was whisked away on my way to the elevator and down the hall to the laboratory for more x-rays, M.R.I. and bone scans plus blood test (C.B.C. B.M.P. C.M.P. MG AND P.S.A.). I came back sometime later and ate a little bit of supper and I was on my way back to the lab for blood work and another scan. I was still down in the laboratory at midnight for still another M.R.I. I returned to my room and got off to sleep at around 1:00 a.m.

I was awakened at 4:30 a.m. by a nurse asking to take my blood, for still a lot more of these tests. About three hours later I had my breakfast brought in, bacon, eggs, toast, jello, coffee and orange juice.

Shortly after breakfast I had my first group of visitors for today. It was my family and my church family. We visited for awhile before Dr. Bourn, an orthopedic surgeon from the Hutchinson Clinic, came in to see me. He looked a little like the Pillsbury Dough Boy. He is a short, blonde headed little roly-poly of a man. After he left I had a real long visit with church friends and family but you know all good things come to an end.

Later on Dr. Fesen and Dr. Bourn came in to talk to me about what they had discovered. They had found a small tumor located somewhere in my neck region. They had a good reason to believe that it could very well be cancerous. Dr. Bourn would become my surgeon. This new finding began to really get to me. Cancer was again a real possibility.

Dr. Bourn ordered more blood tests, scans and M.R.I. He told me he wouldn't be doing any surgery until he could say he was completely sure of and comfortable with what he was going to find when he got in there. Also how he was going to approach the tumor. He came back a few hours later that evening to tell me that he was ready to do the surgery and he would be scheduling it for 9:00 a.m. on the next morning. My P.S.A. had risen now to a huge number of 2900. This meant no food or drink after 12:00 a.m.

This really sent some chills through my whole body. My wife, daughter and granddaughter have been with me from the beginning, also my church family, pastor and his wife have also been with me through it all so far. I thank God for all His blessings.

If this is cancer, this is the disease that killed my mother. She died of colon cancer many many years ago. I have always associated cancer with a very painful death. If I now have cancer and it would seem to be very likely, what was going to happen to me? Was I going to die!!! So many questions and so few answers. Death was something we had never really talked about, but the time had come to talk and do some very serious thinking about it. I guess maybe I am one of those people who has always thought nothing bad like this could ever happen to me. But, now that it has happened to me, where do I go? What do I do about it? Dr. Fesen believes this is going to be prostate cancer that has metastasized to many of the bones in my skeletal system. Having cancer all over my bones definitely is not good at all.

Am I going to die? I have had good friends die from this disease. I knew a young boy eleven years old who died of bone cancer when I was growing up. They kept taking off his limbs. First his lefts, one at a time and so on until his death about one year later. I also have a sister-in-law who has beaten breast cancer. Today she is cancer free for nearly 5 years now. That is, if in fact, we are ever cancer free. Some doctors say we are born with cancer cells in our system that just haven't become active.

MRI CERVICAL SPINE (GENERIC) -
DEITSCH LLOYD
Hutchinson Hospital
Sex: M
ID: 215001
Img [1] #1/12
A
P
F
H
19 cm
DICOM LiteBox 2.70
22 cm
MRI CERVICAL SPINE (GENERIC) -
DEITSCH LLOYD
Hutchinson Hospital
Sex: M
ID: 215001
Img [1] #1/12
A
P
F
H
20 cm
23 cm
MRI CERVICAL SPINE (GENERIC) -
DEITSCH LLOYD
Hutchinson Hospital
Sex: M
ID: 215001
Img [1] #1/12
A
P
F
H
20 cm
23 cm
MRI CERVICAL SPINE (GENERIC) -
DEITSCH LLOYD
Hutchinson Hospital
Sex: M
ID: 215001
Img [1] #1/24
MR - W: 723 L: 318
Pos: 50.375 mm
A
R
L
P
13 cm
DICOM LiteBox 2.70
17 cm

MRI CERVICAL SPINE (GENERIC) -
DEITSCH LLOYD
Hutchinson Hospital
Sex: M
ID: 215001
Img [1] #1/25
MR - W: 1506 L: 681
Pos: 51.924 mm
A
R
L
P
6 cm
DICOM LiteBox 2.70
8 cm
MRI CERVICAL SPINE (GENERIC) -
DEITSCH LLOYD
Hutchinson Hospital
Sex: M
ID: 215001
Img [1] #1/25
MR - W: 1506 L: 681
Pos: 51.924 mm
A
R
L
P
12 cm
DICOM LiteBox 2.70
16 cm
MRI CERVICAL SPINE (GENERIC) -
DEITSCH LLOYD
Hutchinson Hospital
Sex: M
ID: 215001
Img [1] #1/23
MR - W: 663 L: 278
Pos: 42.936 mm
A
R
L
P
12 cm
DICOM LiteBox 2.70
16 cm
MRI CERVICAL SPINE (GENERIC) -
DEITSCH LLOYD
Hutchinson Hospital
Sex: M
ID: 215001
Img [1] #1/25
MR - W: 1510 L: 711
Pos: 28.106 mm
A
R
L
P
13 cm
DICOM LiteBox 2.70
15 cm

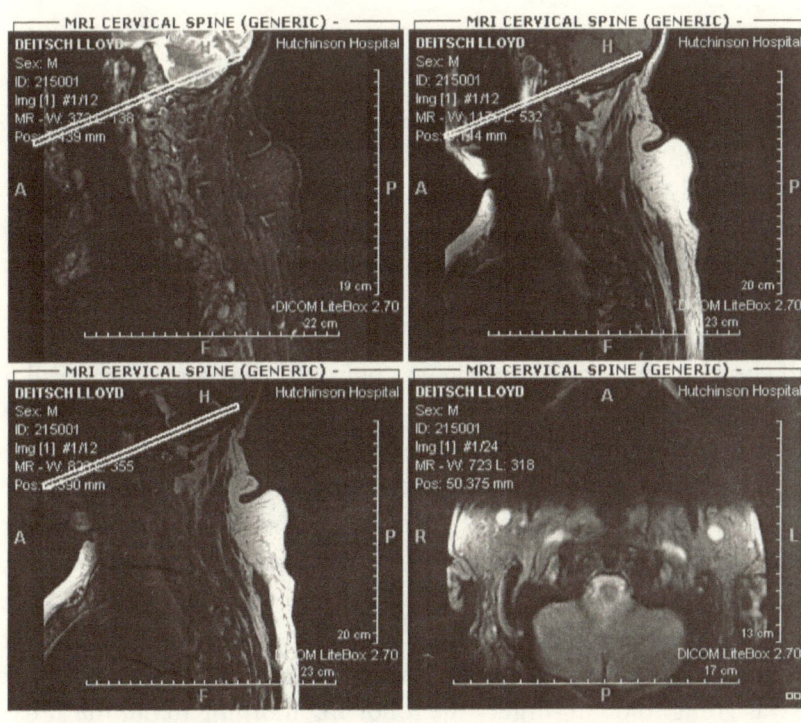

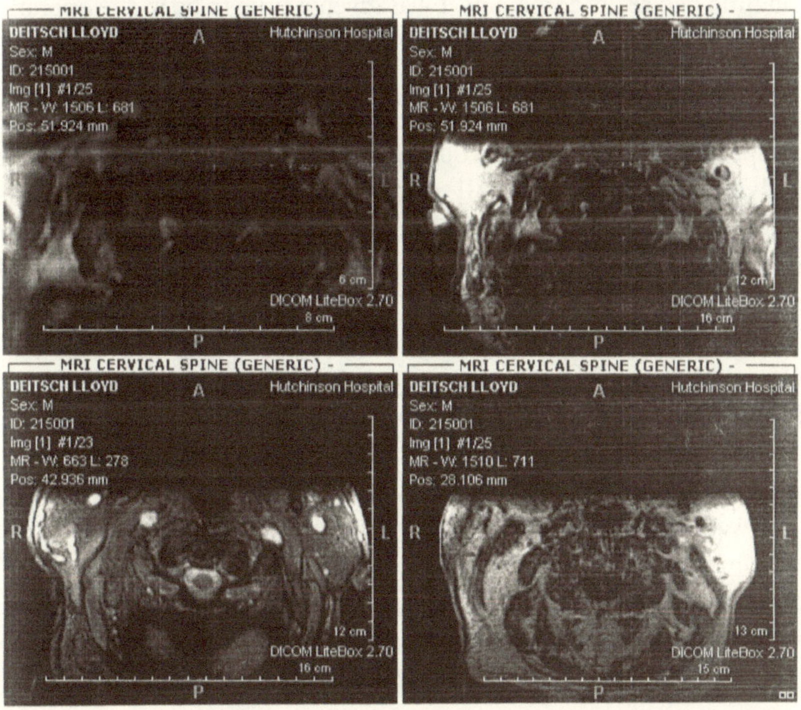

Life is just a precious commodity that we all try very hard to make it last as long as possible, but still many people suffer an awful lot because cancer has gotten them. We don't know from one day to the next what we are going to be doing or even if we are going to be alive. What is coming up for me next, God is the only one that really knows for sure. Believe me it is better that way.

My church operates a religious satellite TV network which sends a signal around the world. It can be found on Dish Satellite systems. The network called Hope Network can be viewed by millions of our friends and church members. My name was put on the air for a prayer call for prayer circles. I don't know who called it in but it appeared on (3ABN) which seems so amazing to me, that my name was going around the world. It makes you feel like there are people out there who really care.

Later in the afternoon as my friends and family are starting to leave, several more doctors came into my room. As the evening was approaching my doctor came in to check me out. I had a heart doctor, an infection doctor, an urologist doctor and my surgeon Dr. Bourn with whom I now have confidence in. Dr. Bourn came to tell me about what he was going to do in surgery the following morning to put me at ease. The time had really come now. I was given a time to be in the operating room at 9:00 a.m. August 25, 2004. He explained to me that I had a small tumor in my neck.

Dr. Bourn said, the tumor itself is located inside the spinal column. It appears to be wrapped around the spinal cord causing me to be paralyzed on my left side. All of this went through my system like a shock. My surgery is going to be in thlke morning. Just a few short hours away. This means no more food or anything to drink after midnight and no breakfast in the morning, *nothing*.

My home church family, who have played a large part in my life have gone home. My friends and my own family, wife, daughter and granddaughter stayed a little while longer. After having a prayer they were all gone for the evening, but they would be back early in the morning before the surgery at 9:00 a.m.

I was all alone now with all my negative thoughts. I had prayed many, many times but nothing like this time. I was worried, I was really scared and I was really upset. My stomach ached. I was what I call a nervous wreck. I had never been in a hospital as a patient before all this started. I was in a strange town, in a strange or unfamiliar surroundings, and now I have cancer and shortly will be having major surgery.

After remembering the Twenty-Third Psalm "The Lord is my shepherd; I shall not want. He maketh me to lie down in green pastures; he leadeth me beside the still waters. He restoreth my soul; he leadeth me in the paths of righteousness for his name's sake. Yes, though I walk through the valley of the shadow of death, I will fear no evil; for thou art with me; thy rod and thy staff they comfort me. Thou preparest a table before me in the presence of mine enemies; thou anointest my head with oil; my cup runneth over. Surely goodness and mercy shall follow me all the days of my life; and I will dwell in the house of the Lord for ever.

Continuing with many hours of intense praying and talking to my Heavenly Father, I had now made peace with my God. I feel sure the Lord will take care of me. My fears were all gone now, and I was very calm and at peace with the world and those who are in it and around me. I was happy.

I don't know for sure when I went to sleep but I was very sure everything was going to be alright and I was very happy when I awakened again at 4:30 a.m. by a nurse who was taking my blood for still another blood test. My (P.S.A.) has now risen to a whopping 2900, but this morning was different though I had never been in this hospital before as a patient, let alone having a major surgery. I was very calm and happily at ease.

I was about to go in for major surgery. I was told to stay in my room and wait for my family to come, along with the pastor and his wife. My two sons who live in the state of Florida will wait at their homes and pray for a successful surgery. It was too short of a notice for them to make the trip in time for the surgery this morning. My family members in Ohio would wait and pray at home.

I was ready now for surgery. I was calm as I continued to wait for family and pastor. As the time approached I began to wonder if they were going to make it in time for the surgery, after all it is some sixty-five miles from my home in Hoisington Kansas.

As 9:00 a.m. arrived on the clock everyone was on time for surgery. At about 9:00 a.m. two Nursing Aides came in and put me on a gurney and took me down to the surgery area to be prepped for surgery. The pastor and my family met for a last prayer circle before going into the operating room to begin my surgery.

I was given my pre-meds and now I was ready to be put on the operating table. This is about to become the biggest adventure of my life. I will now walk through the valley of death. I will fear no evil because Jesus is walking with me and from time to time I am sure of that He may even carry me on my long journey through the valley of the unknown to me.

I do know for sure, that is where the Miracles get started. Now back to my story. I was taken to the operating room and transferred to the operating table. The anesthesiologist came in and gave me a shot and told me to count backwards from one hundred to zero. I think I got to ninety eight more or less. I was now ready for whatever came next. I guess I don't remember seeing any bright lights or tunnel or anything else. The surgery passed so fast and then it was over.

The surgery itself lasted, I was told, from four to four and a half hours, give or take a few minutes. I don't really know for sure. The surgery was performed on the left side of my neck. The fifth cervical vertebra in my neck to be exact.

They opened up my neck by placing an incision on the left side about half way down my neck. They went into the vertebra by going in between and around the veins, arteries and other stuff in this area. This I was told was a very difficult surgery. Dr. Bourn told me the bones were very hard and they needed to be dealt with very carefully so as not to cut something that would cause major problems.

This was the very dangerous part of the surgery. The removing of the tumor without doing any damage to the spinal cord. This area is very small and hard to work on but I had that Great Doctor from up above helping with my surgery. With God anything is possible.

After the Doctors had removed as much of this cancerous tumor as humanly possible, the rest was left for God to take care of, as only He can do. It was now time to put things back together. It was closing time in the operating room.

They couldn't put the same bone piece back in the place it came out of, so they had to replace the bone with cancer on it with a little piece of metal and eight tiny metal screws. The metal piece was made of Titanium (a metal that doesn't cause rejection by the body) and screw it fast to the remaining vertebra to help stabilize the neck.

They also took a small piece of bone from my hip. This piece of bone was to be used as a spacer in the reconstruction of the front side of the fifth vertebra which had a cancerous tumor hooked to it.

My cancer was Prostate in name and it had metastasized onto the many bones in my system, causing it to form a tumor in my neck. We don't know why it stopped there and it didn't go up to the brain, but we are happy it, did not. This makes my cancer a stage four cancer, which is the last stage of cancer. When it leaves its origin and spreads out in my system.

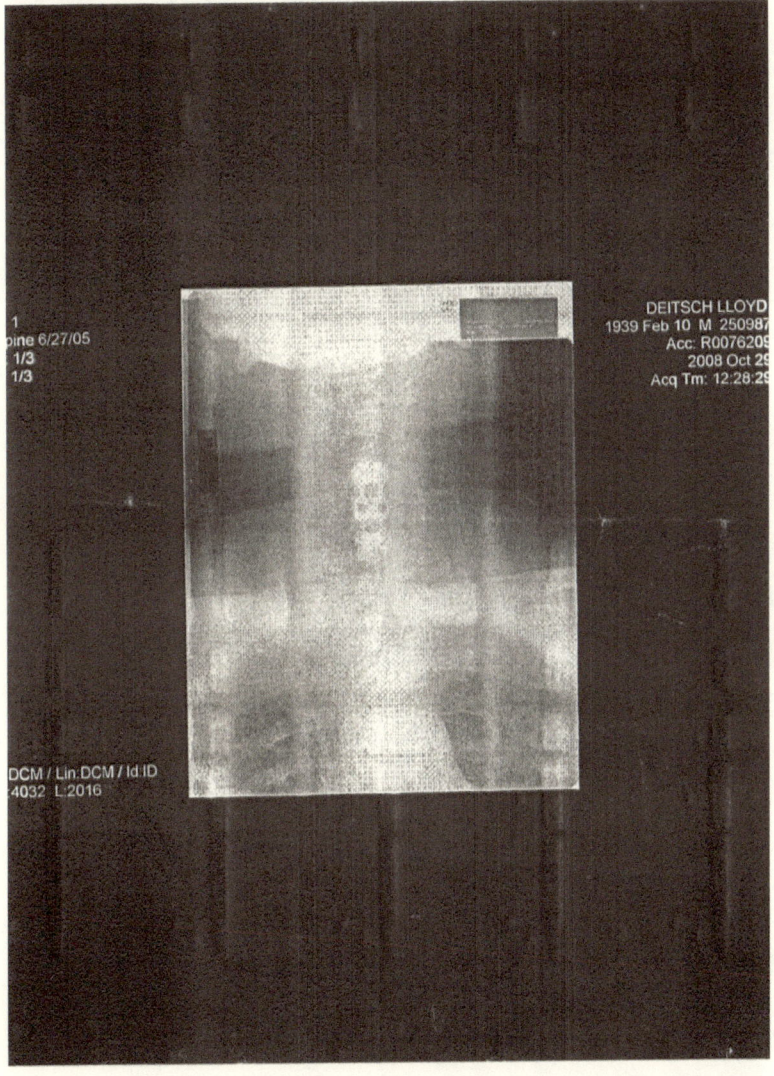

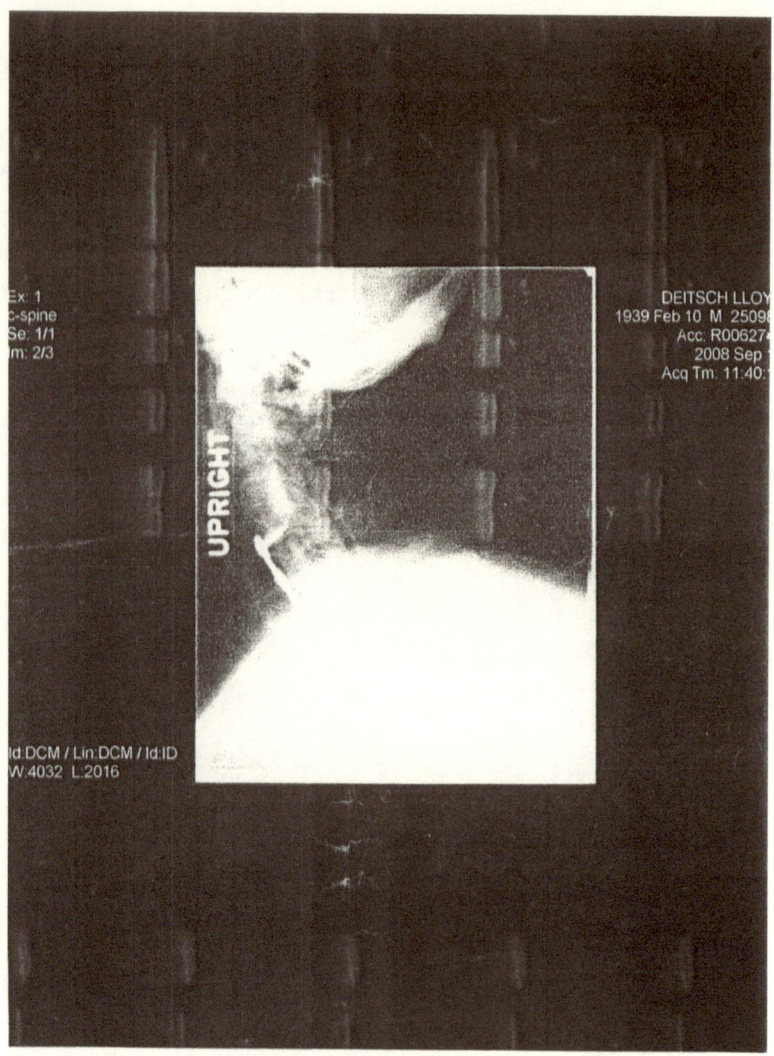

Now back to my story. I was then taken to the recovery room. As I was starting to wake up from surgery, I was beginning to think everything had to have gone very well. I was hearing the voices of my wife, my daughter and granddaughter. The pastor and his wife from church in Great Bend Kansas.

I wasn't in the Intensive Care Unit, I was pretty sure of that. You know the I.C.U. you wouldn't have all of these people in your room. It just wouldn't happen. My wife asked if I was having any pain. I told her I wasn't having any pain after all of this surgery, no pain.

This kind of surgery was supposed to be very painful. This I was told before I went in for surgery. I was also told I would likely never walk again. They said my left arm & leg would likely not be usable as there was a discussion of that possibility. I am beginning to get use to a wheelchair, but not being able to walk, wasn't acceptable to me.

So when I came out of surgery I opened my eyes and saw a gym bar above my head on the bed. I decided to see if I could get a hold on the bar. My brother Don had told me that after surgery I should have my control back. He has had back surgery and he got his control back.

It took just three swings to get a hold of that bar but I did it, I surely did. I could now move my left arm and left leg. I could also use my hand and my fingers. I couldn't hold a baseball or a full cup of coffee but this was a real start.

What a miracle this day is turning out to be for me, my family and my many friends. As my story goes along we will continue to see more and more miracles coming out of this surgery. Everywhere we see the Power of God. I am a firm believer in the Power of Prayer and spending time talking to my God. God's love for us is truly limitless and completely unconditional. If you remember I have had no pain from any of my two surgeries.

I had a very long day so I had a real early night. My friends and family were all gone and on their way home again. With this being my first night after surgery my wife is going to stay all night. I had a large cup of ice and some jello (cherry flavor). I could eat this jello for every meal and there were times when I really did. I love jello.

Dr. Bourn came in to tell me how everything went. I said he wasn't sure that he had gotten all of it. He told me he might have to go back in again at a later time. I was feeling good and nothing he said could change my day and the way I felt. I went off to sleep feeling very content. I was real tired.

The next morning came very early as I was awakened at four thirty by the lab nurse taking my blood for the lab for more testing. I went back to sleep and the next time I woke up it was seven thirty and was time for breakfast. I had a breakfast which included juice, toast, eggs and coffee.

After breakfast a man came into the room to equip me (or fit me) with a neck brace. The equipment had several different kinds of collars to support my neck until it was healed. I will wear this equipment for three to five months.

I also have an oxygen reclaimer to help with my recovery from surgery. I have a breathing machine also to help prevent me from coming down with pneumonia. This is a major problem for people who are recovering from major surgery.

Now back to my story. A P.T. Tech (Physical Therapist) came into the room to get me out of bed, to see if I can walk. That was a real joke, don't you know. The R.P.M.S. my room was spinning, was great. I was put in a chair for dinner while my bed was being changed. My P.S.A. had now dropped down to 7.04. But this still is too high to live with. It needed to be below 4.4. Anything more than that is really too high.

So they decided to do more surgery. I will be having my testicles removed. This surgery was performed by still another surgeon by the name of Dr. Wingart. I never became too friendly with him. I still had no pain yet with any of my surgeries. Some of the doctors are calling me their miracle patient. It seems like everything is going very well. Maybe I will be able to return to Great Bend soon.

My lat lab test now shows that my P.S.A. has dropped down to 0.00, which is very good. I am very pleased with my P.S.A. What does P.S.A. really stand for? I have no idea.

I have had many visitors today coming and going all day long. Tonight for supper I will be having roast beef, potatoes and gravy, peas and my favorite jello. It was a really good mean but not like homemade. Hospital food is just not up to par. They came and took my oxygen reclaimer away tonight but that was okay with me, because I wasn't using it anyway. I have only used it two times since I had surgery.

The third night after my second surgery a nurse came and told me I was getting a blood transfusion this evening. I waited all evening and it never happened. So I got ready to go to sleep. Guess what! Here comes my blood.

At eleven thirty P.M. here comes my blood. The nurse came in with two bags of packed cells. It was started at, straight up midnight and would take four full hours. Needless to say, I wouldn't need to be awakened at four-thirty A.M. for a blood test. I will be awake. Who can sleep with a board taped to their arm. Well, it was over at four ten or four fifteen.

I had finally gotten through with my blood work and my oxygen. Which I haven't had for days. My breathing machine and two of my heparin locks, so I thought I was doing pretty good. I looked out the window and down below me was what resembled a small race track. I asked the Doctor what that was for. He told me I had to be able to walk all the way around that track before I can go back to Great Bend. I asked who he was kidding because if that was the case, I will be a permanent resident because I can't walk six feet without a walker. He later told me they used that track for knee replacement patients.

We are continuing to have prayer circles daily. Asking God to heal me from the dreaded disease. Eight days now after I went to the Hutchinson Hospital for major surgery. I am now returning to the local hospital in Great Bend (C.K.M.C. Central Kansas Medical Center) for in-hospital physical therapy, so now I am returning home so to speak.

My daughter drove me home back to Great Bend to the hospital in my car. Medicare won't pay for transfers between hospitals if it isn't absolutely a necessity. I guess I could have stayed in Hutchinson and my family do all the driving. Not a good idea. When checking into the hospital. I was tired after putting things away and getting settled in. I ate my supper and then I went to bed early that night. It was good to be home.

The next day I began physical therapy in the morning as an inpatient. After breakfast I had a lot of things to learn before I would be allowed to return to my home in Hoisington Kansas. I had to be able to transfer myself from wheelchair to the bed and back to chair. I also had to be able to go to the restroom and transfer to stool and back to chair. Later I had a large group of visitors from church. I always enjoy my visitors. The more visitors the merrier. I also need to learn the mechanics of my wheelchair, Lock The Wheels.

I am now getting my grip back a little at a time in my left hand. I now have forty-one pounds in my right hand and twenty-one pounds in my left hand. When I left Hutchinson my grip was three pounds in my left hand. I have been working very hard to build up my left side. I am working with a physical therapist tech at Great Bend Hospital (C.K.M.C.). No more forty-thirty A.M. wakeup calls by a nurse wanting more blood for testing.

About two weeks or fifteen days later, we made a short visit to my home in Hoisington to see what we needed to have done before I could return home. We needed a ramp for a wheelchair which we already had done. I needed a bath chair which we already had. We had the ramp built by a church member before I went to the hospital.

Early this morning, after my visit I was getting my things together, packing my case and bag for my trip home. Now all I could do was wait for my daughter to take me home, after three and a half weeks at Hutchinson and Great Bend Hospitals. I was now on my way home by car. By the way, my grip had improved to thirty pounds of grip in my left hand. I had already built up my muscle tone in my arms and legs. I could pump 200 pounds with my left and my right leg.

Now back to my story. Again the first week in October, the sixth to be exact. I met with Dr. Fesen at the Heartland Cancer Center in Great Bend, Kansas. I am now scheduled for a CT and a bone scan at C.K.M.C. in Great Bend for eight A.M. on Thursday, October 7, 2004. I need an injection of dye for this scan. I had already had a blood test.

For the month of October 2004, my blood tests this month will be at C.K.M.C. on Mondays as follows:

October 11, 18, & 25 C.B.C. B.M.P. on the 18th a P.S.A. My new P.S.A. was 0.006.

October 13 I saw Dr. Fesen and he sent me to see Dr. Prez DaMilo who started radiation that very day. I was scheduled for radiation on the 13, 14, 15, 19, 20, 21, 22, 26, 27, 29 and 29th, also I saw Dr. Fesen on the 13, 20, and 27th and his P.A. Lorrie on the 22nd. This was one busy month for me.

The radiation was focused on my neck and on the spot where the tumor was removed. I had to have pre-meds in the chemo room of the Heartland cancer. I would go in and set down. the nurses would threat a needle in the back of my hand for meds. Sometimes the fluid lines would become plugged and or just stopped. Then we would start all over again. But these meds are a real help to prevent side effects.

The many pre-meds took sometimes almost two hours to complete. The radiation itself takes maybe five minutes to do on the radiation table. This treatment would make my neck swell. The swelling would cause a lot of trouble in swallowing food or drinking water. It would get so sore and there wasn't much you could do about it. It has been about four months since I had surgery. My rehabilitation with my arm and leg is going along very well. My P.S.A. is down to 0.000 and that is very good. Everything as we look over the year 2004 is definitely improving.

In the month of November it was getting cool outside. In November my labs were taken at C.K.M.C. on the 8, 15, 22 and 29th. My outpatient physical therapy on the eighth of November, 2004 and continued on the 10, 11, 15, 16, 17, 20, 24, 26, 29 and 30th. My radiation continued on November 2, 3, 4, 5, 9, and 16th and this completed my radiation treatments. I also saw Dr. Fesen on November 10, 2004.

On the first day of December I had a visit with Dr. Fesen and got my chemotherapy scheduled for three hours a day one day a week, but before I started chemo I had a port inserted into my right chest area. My Doctor for this surgery was Dr. Kerby from Great Bend. The surgery was performed at C.K.M.C. in Great Bend. A port is about the size of a quarter and is covered by a rubbery substance which will let a needle be inserted for chemo. The port is connected to a vein. This is why you can gain access to a vein with a needle stick.

My blood work was done at Hutchinson Clinic on December the sixth because I had an appointment, my first since my surgery, with Dr. Bourn for a checkup on my neck surgery. I am still wearing the brace. I hope, maybe, I will be able to get it off. I am getting two x-rays of my neck. He isn't happy with what he is seeing. The bones in my neck are not knitting together as they should be. So I won't be getting rid of my brace.

He also checked my knee and my arm. He said things were getting better but, he still doesn't think I will ever walk again and that I should be very happy in my wheelchair for the rest of my life. I sure didn't like that idea at all.

The other labs were drawn at C.K.M.C. on December 13, 20 and 27th. My physical therapist dates this month are 2, 3, 4, 7, 9, 10, 13, 14, 16, 20, 21, 23 and the 27th. Fourteen physical therapy days this month. I hope the New Year will be better than this past year. First I was scheduled for sixteen radiation treatments and now chemo once a week. I asked Dr. Fasen what my chances are. He told me that maybe he could buy me some time. This wasn't exactly what I wanted to hear but it was better than thirty, sixty or ninety days.

Christmas this year, hasn't been a very merry season, but at least we are all still together. We pray things will get better with time.

HAPPY NEW YEAR 2005
SPECIMEN INQUIRY
HEMATOLOGY

Complete Blood Count

W.B.C.	5.0		4.0-10.8	k/mm-3
R.B.C.	4.2	L	4.5-5.9	m/mm-3

Hemoglobin & Hematocrit

Hemoglobin	13.6	13.6-17.5	k/mm-3
Hematocrit	40.5	40-54	m/mm-3
M.C.V.	96	80-100	gm/1
M.C.H.	32.5	26-34	%
M.C.H.C.	33.7	32.36	f/
R.D.W.	15.6	12-16	pg
Platelet Count	247	150-350	k/mm-3
M.P.V.	7.0	7-9	f/
Neutrophils	58.5	42.62	%
Lymphocyte	28.2	20-51	%

Monocytes	9.3		1.7-9.3	%
Eosinophil	3.7		0.7-7	%
Basophil	9.3	H	0-0.2	%
Neutrophils #	2.93		1.4-6.5	
Lymphocyte #	1.41		1.2-3.4	
Monocyte #	0.47		0.1-0.6	
Eosinophil #	0.19		0-0.7	
Basophils #	0.02		0-0.2	k/mm-3

SPECIMEN INQUIRY
CHEMISTRY

Basic Metabolic Profile

Glucose	115	H	74-106	mg/dL
Bun	13		7-18	mg/dL
Creatinine Serum	0.9		0.6-1.5	mg/dL
Bun & Creatinine Ratio	14.00		6-2600	
Sodium	140		135-155	meg/L
Potassium	3.6		3.5-5.1	meg/L
Chloride	103		98-107	meg/L
Carbon Dioxide	33.7	H	21-32	mmol/L
Calcium Level	8.6		8.5-10.1	mg/dL
Total Protein	6.1		6.4-8.2	mg/dL
Albumin	4.1		3.4-5.0	gm/L
Globulin	2.6		2.4-3.5	gm/L
Osmolality	287		261-287	gml
Albumin/Globulin Ratio	1.6		1.1-2.2	
Bilirubin Total	0.2		0.2-1.0	u/L

AST/SGOT	24	15-37	u/L
Magnesium Level	1.9	1.8-2.4	mg/L
Alkaline Phosphatase	117	42-128	u/L
ALT/SGPT	50	30-65	u/L

SPECIAL CHEMISTRY

P.S.A. Diagnostic	0.000	0.1-4.1	n/L
	40	0.1-1.4	
	40-50	0.1-2.0	
	50-60	0.1-3.1	
	60-70	0.1-4.1	
	70	0.1-4.4	

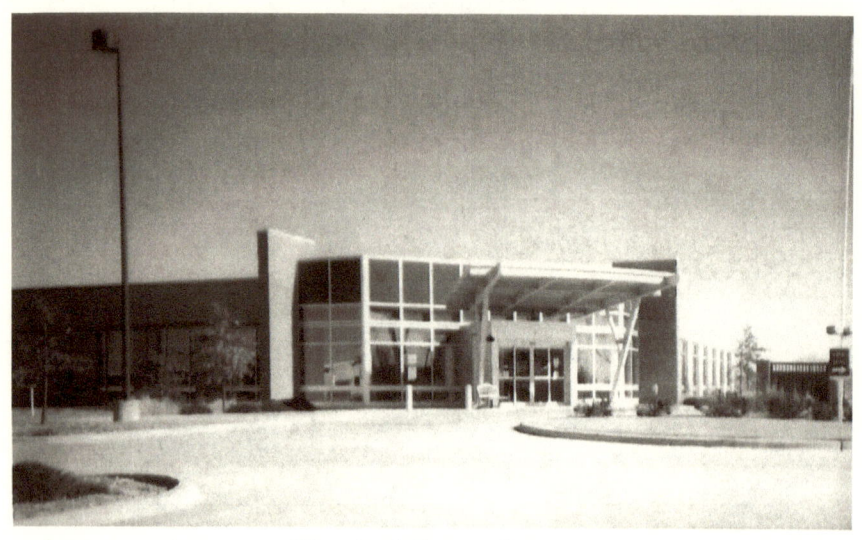

Heartland Cancer Center

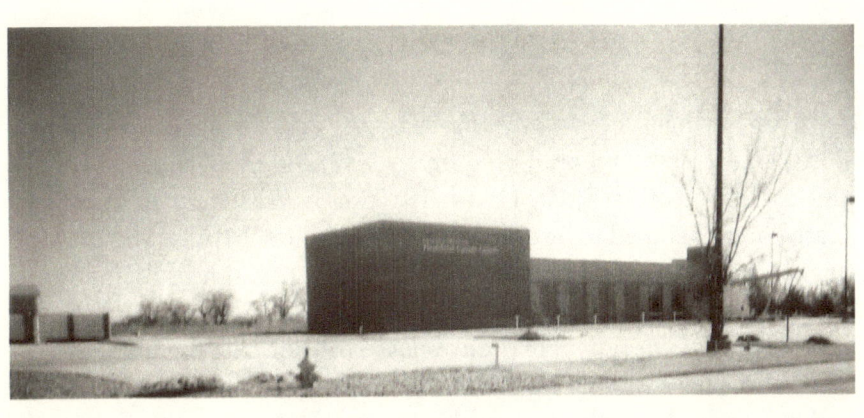

HAPPY NEW YEAR

2005

A New Year to start my labs. I will continue my labs for January on 3, 10, 17, 24 and 31st. This was a very quiet month not much really going on. My physical therapy this month are on 4, 6, 7, 10, 11, 13, 17, 18, 20, 24, 26, 28, and 31st. My physical therapy is now. I am making progress on my walking rehabilitation. I am seeing Dr. Fesen on the 12th. I am taking two chemotherapies by the name of Taxol and Cabopatine. All my labs will be completed at the hospital in Great Bend, C.K.M.C. this month.

FEBRUARY 2005

I am having a visit with Dr. Fesen on the 2nd and again on February 23rd. Dr. Fesen says I am doing pretty well. My physical therapy days this month are 1, 4, 7, 10, 11, 14, 18, 21, 23, 25, and 28th. Taxol and Carbo are scheduled to be done on 2, 16, and 23rd. My labs will be done at the Great Bend Hospital on the 7, 14, 21, and 28th of the month. I also had a second visit with Dr. Bourn. He still isn't satisfied with the way my neck is healing. He didn't release me nor take the brace away.

I also have a birthday this month on the 10th. I didn't do too much today. I truly didn't think I would live to see this day. Dr. Fesen said he could buy me some time but didn't tell me how much. I did have physical therapy today. I am trying to learn to walk again and I can't even see my feet or the floor because of the brace on my neck. The weather was cold and very damp but no snow. I suppose it could have been a lot worse.

MARCH 2005

The month of March was a busy one. My labs were on the 6, 13, 20, and 27th at Great Bend Hospital. My chemo day starts with seeing Dr. Fesen. Then I have 1 to 1½ hours of pre-meds, 1 hour of magnesium and 3 hours of chemo, Taxol and Cabopatin a total of 4½ to 5½ hours. I have chemo on the 2, 9, and 23rd.

On the fourth I had a C.T. scan at the hospital in the Great Bend C.K.M.C. I check in the hospital at 2:15 for paperwork before having my scan at 2:30 P.M. I have to report into the hospital at 10:30 A.M. for a shot of dye injected into my veins and then come back in the afternoon for the bone scan. It didn't take very long. Overall, this takes about an hour. On the 25th or the day after is my bone scan. I have an M.R.I. at the Great Bend hospital C.K.M.C. it was scheduled for 7:30 A.M.

These scans are being done to show how many white spots are still on my skeletal system. All of my labs will now be drawn in Hoisington at C.B.H. Clara Barton Hospital. We continue to pray for a quick cure. My family and church family continues to pray. They call on the phone and we see them in church regularly for support. March has been a very busy month.

APRIL 2005

In the month of April things were basically the same. I have my blood drawn on the 4, 11, 18, and 25th at Hoisington, Kansas at C.B.H. My chemos are the same as last month. The days are the 6, 13, and 27th. I saw Dr. Fesen on the second and fourth Wednesday or twice a month.

MAY 2005

In the month of May I had chemo three to four hours a day on the 4, 18, and 25th at the Heartland Cancer in Great Bend. My labs this month will be drawn in Hoisington at C.B.H. on the 2, 9, 16, 23, and 30th. The blood tests are namely C.B.C., B.M.P., C.M.P., Mg and a P.S.A. What do all these letters mean? I have no idea. We continue to pray for healing.

JUNE 2005

In June I have my blood drawn in Hoisington on the 6, 13, 20, and 27th at C.B.H. I have my chemo on the 8, 15, and 29th. I am having chemo three weeks on and one week off. I saw Dr. Fasen twice this month. My blood test this week of 27 was drawn at Hutchinson at the clinic. I have to see Dr. Bourn, my surgeon for a checkup. He took my neck brace away but didn't release me. He wanted to know how I was dealing with the idea of not being able to walk. I didn't tell him that I could walk. I have one more visit with him at least.

JULY 2005

The month of July was a real quiet month. My blood was drawn at the hospital in Hoisington on the 5, 11, 18, and 25th. My chemos are on 6, 20, and 27th of this month at the Heartland Cancer Center. The weather outside was now starting to get very hot and dry. The grass has all turned brown. No more grass to mow. I continue to improve as time goes on.

AUGUST 2005

In the month of August I am scheduled to have an (E.C.H.O.) Gram. On Thursday I went to have this done to check my heart. At the Clara Barton Hospital. This hospital is a very good one for being in a small town of less than 4000 population. I am also having a cervical scan of my neck on the third of the month on Wednesday at 10:45 A.M. at (C.K.M.C.).

All my labs this month will be drawn at the hospital in Hoisington C.B.H. on the (1, 8, 15, 22, and 29th). My chemos this month will be on the (10, 24, and 31st). All of my chemos this month will be administered at the Heartland Cancer Center in Great Bend, Kansas.

26

It has been a full year since I was diagnosed with a cancerous tumor. After finding a tumor in my neck and then having surgery, by Dr. Bourn, he removed the tumor.

My chemos are on the 7, 21, and 28th of the month. My blood was drawn on the 5, 12, 19 and 26th of the month. I also have an appointment to see Dr. Youngman at 1:00 P.M. on September 6, at the Clara Barton Clinic in Hoisington, Kansas.

Dr. Youngman is checking my (E.C.H.O.) gram for congestive heart failure. He told me my heart was in good shape for my age. The (E.C.H.O.) gram is done by putting a jelly liquid on my chest and stomach. They use a magnetic probe on my chest and stomach and it transmits a signal to a computer screen that shows any heart problems. I am very glad that I didn't have any heart problems. I also have mag on (6, 7,8, 9, 13, 16, 20, 21, 28, and 30th). My mag was very very low. We continue to pray for strength and also for healing. I really need the prayers of everyone.

I made a trip to see Dr. Bourn on the 19th of September. I wasn't really satisfied with him. He kept telling me I will never walk again. So I took my wheelchair with me. I had two x-rays and he examined me. He said I was doing very well and released me. He then turned and walked out of the room. I got out of my wheelchair and walked out behind him. When he saw me I got a big laugh. I wish I would have had a camera. The look on his face was priceless. The bones in my neck were all knitted and there wasn't any sign of the tumor. Praise God.

We thank God for His blessing. We continue to pray for a quick recovery and an end to the chemo. People don't believe in miracles today but I do. My church and my belief in God have been a big source of strength for me through this disease and the treatment which I have been receiving.

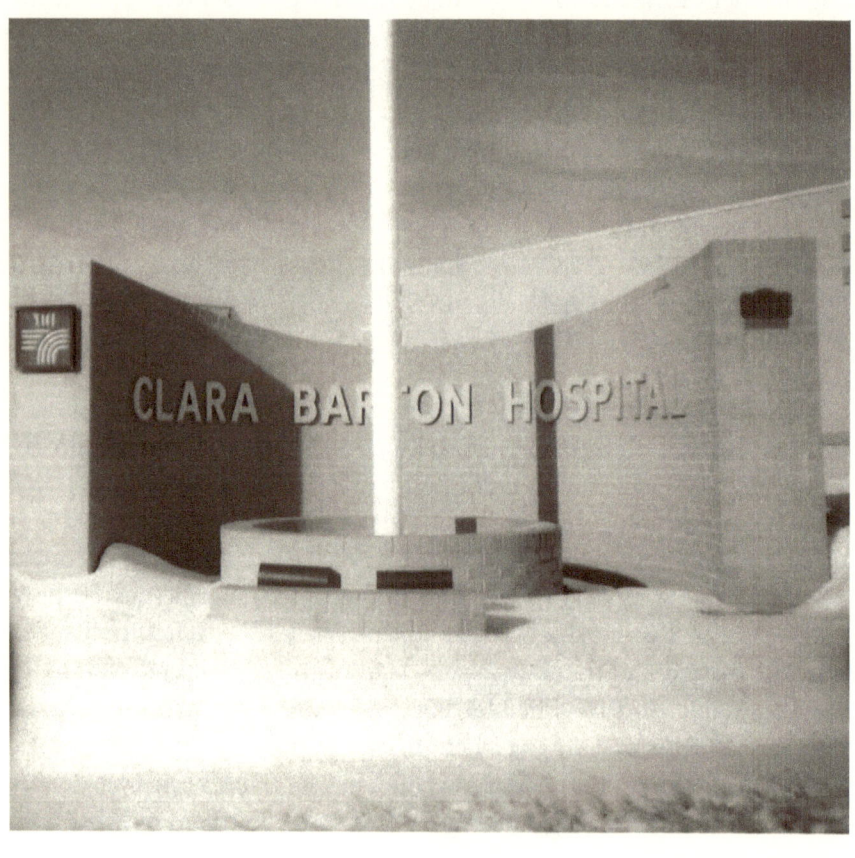

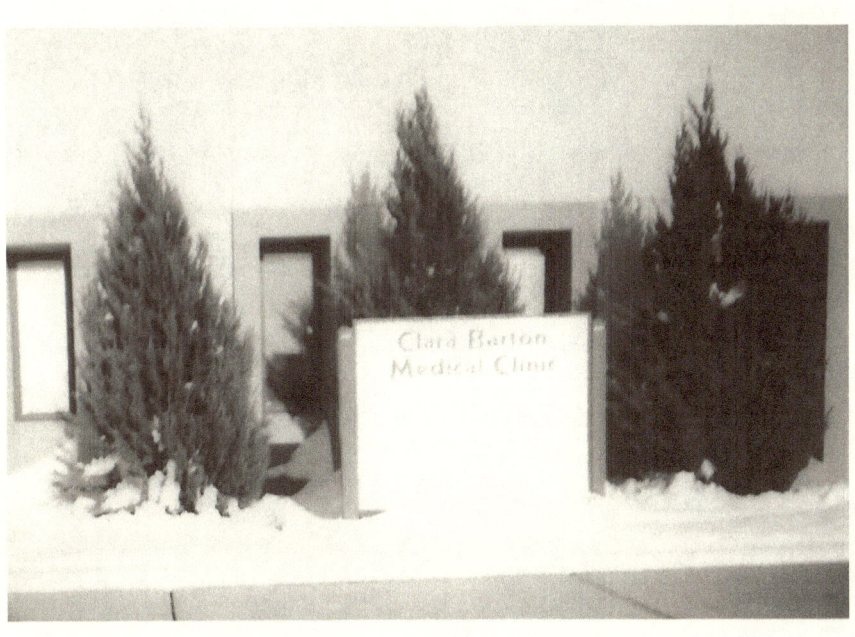

Linked Items:

MRI CERV W/O CONT on 03/10/2006 1148 Order/Occ: X340345-1

Order Phys: FESEN,MARK R Order Dx: 185—MALIGN NEOPL PROSTA

Reason For Exam?" CA PROSTATE

MRI LUMB W&W/O CONT on 03/03/2006 0707 Order/Occ: X339475-1

Order Phys: FESEN,MARK R Order Dx: 185—MALIGN NEOPL PROSTA

Reason For Exam?: CA PROSTATE

MRI THOR W&W/O CONT on 03/03/2006 0707 Order/Occ: X339475-1

Order Phys: FESEN,MARK R Order Dx: 185—MALIGN NEOPL PROSTA

Reason For Exam?" CA PROSTATE

CERVICAL, THORACIC AND LUMBAR SPINE MRI

HISTORY: Prostate CA.

This examination was completed over several days worth of scanning. The patient was unable to tolerate the entire examination being performed in one day. Essentially the pre-contrast studies were completed on 03/03/06. The final post contrast studies were not completed until 03/10/06.

COMPARISON EXAMINATION: MRI from 11/16/.05

MRI CERVICAL SPINE: The cervical spine MRI is of marginal diagnostic quality. There are postoperative changes in the mid cervical spine with anterior fusion of C4, C5 and C6. This anterior fusion plate is producing significant artifact through this area. The cervical vertebral bodies are riddled with heterogeneous signal consistent with metastatic involvement. The patient has not developed any compression fractures. The transaxial images show spondylosis at multiple levels. It would be very difficult to assess for any significant stenosis due to the artifact secondary to the postoperative changes in the mid cervical spine and quality of the images.

MRI OF THE THORACIC SPINE: Again the vertebral bodies of the thoracic spine are mottled with heterogeneous signal intensity, all consistent with metastatic involvement. No pathologic compression fractures have developed since the previous examination. No significant stenosis is appreciated. The examination is stable from the prior study.

IMRESSION:

Stable thoracic spine MRI with riddling of multiple vertebral bodies, consistent with metastatic involvement. No pathologic compression fractures.

MRI OF THE LUMBAR SPINE: The marrow signal of the lumbar spine is very heterogeneous in signal, consistent with metastatic involvement. Multilevel degenerative disc disease is again noted. There are multilevel spondylosis changes with some stenosis at L3-4 and particularly L4-5 due to the degenerative spondylosis change. No compression fractures have developed since the previous study.

IMPRESSION:
1. Stable moderate appearance of the lumbar vertebral bodies, consistent with metastatic involvement. There is no indication of any pathologic fractures.
2. There is spinal canal, lateral recess and neural foraminal stenosis, most severe at L4-5. This is secondary to marked degenerative changes and spondylosis.
3. The lumbar spine is not significantly changed from the comparison study.

Dictated By: WILSON,GARY L DO 03/10/2006 1325
Released By: (Electronic Signature) SIGNED
WILSON,GARY L DO 03/11/2006 0728
Transcribed: ETR 03/10/2006 1524

Signed by: Signed at:

X-Ray

Patient: Jr Lloyd Deitsch   EMRN: 250987
           221 N Green St   Age/DOB: 69/Feb 10, 1939

           Hoisington, KS 67544
                                        Home: (620)617-7150
Encounter Date: Dec 6 2004 12:00AM   Work:

DEITSCH, LLOYD   A-250987   (X-RAY)

12/06/2004—INTERPRETATION OF RADIOGRAPHS: Cervical
spine AP and lateral x-rays, December 6, 2004.

   DESCRIPTION: Cervical C5 corpectomy and anterior fusion has
been performed. Tibial allograft is in excellent position. There are no
lucencies adjacentto the cervical C4 and C6-7 plates. Anterior plate
contour is appropriate. There are no lucencies adjacent to the fixation
screws. There are no fractures.

   IMPRESSION: Cervical C5 corpectomy and anterior fusion
                      with plating.

                 Samuel M. Bourn, MD/emw

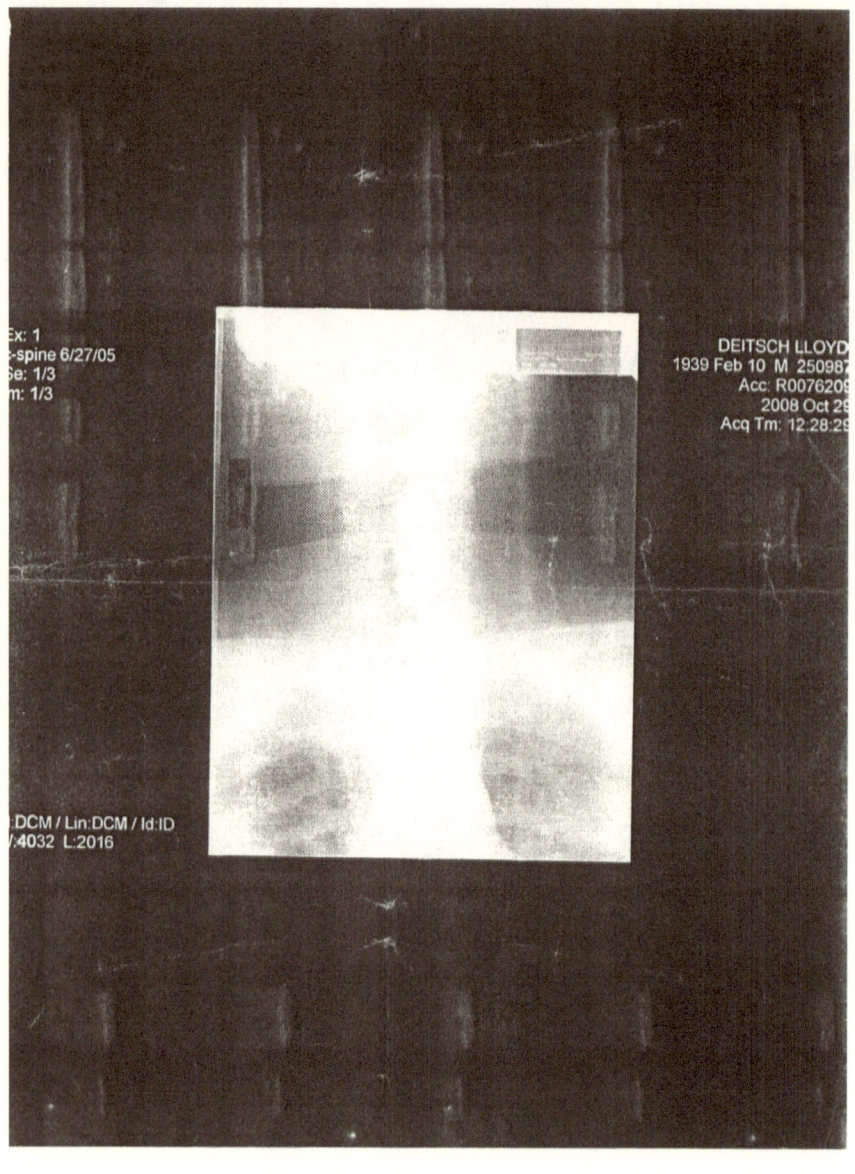

Ex: 1
x-spine 6/27/05
Se: 1/3
m: 1/3

DEITSCH LLOYD
1939 Feb 10 M 250987
Acc: R0076209
2008 Oct 29
Acq Tm: 12:28:29

:DCM / Lin:DCM / Id:ID
W:4032 L:2016

I also have a very strong belief in my Doctor and the nursing staff that treat me every week at the Heartland Cancer Center. This staff, the many hospitals and many clinics I have been to up to date.

OCTOBER 2005

Now we move on to the month of October. Fall is coming. The leaves are brown and are falling off the trees. There is a chill in the air. I am starting to get zometa this month. It is given intravenously to help with the bones and skeletal system. It really helps your bones feel better, but it just lasts for a few days at a time.

I have my labs drawn this month on (3, 10, 15, 24, and 31st). On the 31st I have a (TSH, C.B.C., C.M.P., Mg, P.T. and P.S.A. tests). My chemos this month are on the (5, 12, and 19th) also on the 19th I have a (P.F.T.) test. I think this is a bone density test. I have no idea what some of these letters stand for.

Over this year I have lost some real good friend but me. I continue to have a real good outlook or frame of mind. I have been asked by several people, people about my cancer because they say I don't act like someone who has cancer. I asked them how a person with cancer is suppose to act. I like to laugh and have a good time, it makes me feel good. You know you have cancer so why feel down if you don't have to.

NOVEMBER 2005

It is now November 11. We have cold weather but no snow as of yet, but it can't be far down the line. I have an eye appointment at Dr. Harold's old office, of course Dr. Harold is no longer with us. I see Dr. Fesen on November 2nd for a checkup up see how I am doing and check my lungs. I have my labs drawn in Hoisington on (7, 14, 21 and 28th) of this month. I have my chemo on the (2, 9 and 23rd). I also have (zometa) on the 2nd of the month. I am still taking two kinds of chemo, (Taxol and Carbopatine).

On the 4th I have an appointment with Dr. Oharia at (C.K.M.C.) at 1:30 P.M. for a sleep test. After talking to her I cancelled it. She said I had to go to Wichita for the test. I wasn't going to Wichita. On the 10th at 8:30 A.M. I have a (M.R.I.) scheduled at (advanced imaging), next door to the cancer center. on the 11th I have a (C.T.) scan at (C.K.M.C.) Kansas Medical Center at 7:30 A.M.

On the 15th of November I have a dentist appointment to have my teeth pulled. Chemo is very hard on your teeth. Bad teeth cause yeast infection in your mouth which does down to your lungs, and believe me you don't want yeast infection in your lungs.

DECEMBER 2005

The month of December is a very slow month. No big exam to be done, no (C.T., or M.R.I.) but still have my labs drawn. I did start taking (Neulasta) shot each time I have chemo for energy and it keeps me from being run down. I have my chemo the (14 and 28th). I am now taking chemo twice a month. My labs are drawn on the (5, 12, 19 and 28th) of this month. I see Dr. Fesen on the 14th.

It is Christmas time this year. When we celebrate the birth of Christ. I pray daily, thanking God for all His Blessings and we ask for his care in getting over this disease.

HAPPY NEW YEAR 2006

This is now January 2006. I will be getting zometa for my aching bones. We hope the New Year will bring new hope for a speedy recovery. God works in many different ways. We pray a lot with my church, friends and family. The Bible says we are never given more than we can bear.

I am now taking a pill, Casadex. This med helps keep the cancerous cells down. I am taking chemo twice a month. In January on the (11 and 25th). My labs are still being drawn on Monday. This month on (2, 9, 16, 23 and 30th). I had a visit with Dr. Fesen for a checkup. I guess I am doing okay.

After one year and five months of chemo and radiation. I can now walk and I can use my arm and hand. I am happy, but I do still have cancer to deal with. I pray often that this disease, cancer will soon be over.

FEBRUARY 2006

Today is the first day of February and is also the day that I see Dr. Fesen for my checkup. Today I also have chemo and mg on the 15th of this month.

My labs are being drawn on the (6, 13, 20 and 27th). As usual at Clara Barton Hospital. My labs are (C.B.C., B.M.P. and P.S.A.). I have having another birthday, the big 67. We didn't do anything special this year. Just stayed home and had green chili for supper. This is my second birthday since they found out that I had cancer.

Empowering Healthcare

Reason For Exam?" CA PROSTATE, SPINE METS

LUMBAR SPINE MRI:

The lumbar spine was scanned in multiplanar, multisequence images pre and post gadolinium administration.

HISTORY: CA of prostate with spine metastases.

COMPARISON STUDY

FINDINGS: Today's evaluation again shows a heterogeneous signal intensity to the marrow structures of the lower thoracic, lumbar spine and upper sacrum. This is all consistent with diffuse metastatic involvement with no interval progression since the previous examination. The patient has not developed any pathologic fractures. All the disk spaces are desiccated. There is acquired stenosis that is stable at L4-5 and L5-S1 secondary to spondylosis and facet hypertrophy.

IMPRESSION
1. Stable lumbar spine MRI, there is diffuse heterogeneous signal that is present in the vertebral bodies and the sacrum is consistent with diffuse metastatic disease without progression.
2. No pathologic fractures.
3. Moderate acquired stenosis at L4-5 and L5-s1, secondary to spondylosis.

Dictated By: WILSON, GARY L DO
Released By: (Electronic Signature) SIGNED
WILSON, GARY L DO

Signed by: Signed at:

MARCH 2006

In March we were a little busier. I see Dr. Fasen on the 7 and 29th. I had my chemo on the 8th of this month. My labs were drawn on the (6, 13, 20 and 27th). On the 9th I had a (C.T. C/A/P). I checked in at 8:15 A.M. and the (C.T.) was done at 9:00. I also have another bone scan. Checkin time at 10:30 for a dye injection. The scan will be done later this afternoon at about 1:00 P.M. All of these tests will be done at the Hospital in Great Bend C.K.M.C. Central Kansas Medical Center where most of my scans are done. I also have a (M.R.I.) at 7:30 A.M. on Friday the third of March. On the 27th my labs test showed that my (P.S.A.) had climbed to 0.245 range. The normal range should be between 0.1 to 4.1.

When I had my surgery in August a year and six months ago, I was on blood pressure medication. My blood pressure was very high. Since surgery my blood pressure is averaging 126 over 76 which is normal. I don't know what happened exactly but it must have been good.

APRIL 2006

In April my monthly appointments were down. I am still doing just one chemo a month. I see Dr. Fesen just once this month and have my chemo on the 5th of April. My labs are going to be drawn on (3, 10, 17 and 24th), at the Clara Barton Hospital in Hoisington, Kansas. There is no (P.S.A.) this month. I don't know why.

SPECIMEN INQUIRY
HEMATOLOGY

Complete Blood Count

W.B.C.	7.0		4.8-10.6	k/mm-3
R.B.C.	4.09	L	4.5-5.9	m/mm-3

Hemoglobin & Hematocrit

Hemoglobin	13.5		13.5-17.5	gm/L
Hematocrit	40.2		40-54	%
M.C.V.	98		80-100	f/L
M.C.H.	330		26-34	pg
M.C.H.C.	33.5		32-36	g/d:
R.D.W.	222		150-350	k/mm-3
M.P.V.	7.2		7-9	f1
Neutrophils	66.3	H	42-62	%
Lymphocyte	24.0		20-51	%
Monocytes	6.5		1.7-93	%
Eosinophil	2.7	H	0-7	%
Basophil	0.5		0-2.0	%

Neutrophils #	4.61	1.4-6.5
Lymphocyte #	1.61	1.2-3.4
Monocytes #	0.45	0.1-.06
Eosinophil #	0.19	0-0.7
Basophil #	0.03	0-0.2 k/mm-3

SPECIMEN INQUIRY
CHEMISTRY

Basic Metabolic Profile

Glucose	105		74-106	mg/dL
Bun	11		7-18	mg/dL
Creatinin Serum	0.9		0.1-1.3	mg/dL
Bun/Creatinin Ratio	12.00		6.00-2600	mg/dL
Sodium	141		135-155	meg/dL
Potassium	4.0		3.5-5.1	meg/dL
Chloride	10.2		98-107	mg/L
Carbon Dioxide	32.0		21-32	mg/L
Calcium Level	8.6		8.5-10.1	mg/L
Osmolality	281	H	261-280	mg/L
Total Protein	6.7		6.4-8.2	gm/dL
Albumin	4.1		3.4-5.0	gm/dL
Globulin	2.6		2.4-3.5	gm/dL
Albumin/Globulin Ratio	1.6		1.1-2.2	go5m/k3
Bilirubin Total	0.2		0.2-1.0	mg/dL

AST/SGOT	24	15-37 u/L
Magnesium Level	1.9	1.8-2.4 mg/dL
Alkaline Phosphatase	117	42-128 u/L
ALT/SGPT	50	30-65 u/L

MAY 2006

I have many changes coming in this month. On the third of May I see Dr. Fesen and took four hours of chemo and pre-meds.

My labs continue to be drawn at Clara Barton Hospital, on the 1, 8, 15, 22, and 29th. I had my P.S.A. run on the first of this month. It has now risen to .650. Dr. Fesen said I had some mutient cancer cells that have found a way to get around the chemo. So we have a new approach coming up, but before we do lets go back to my physical therapy days at the hospital in Great Bend as an out patient.

MY PHYSICAL THERAPY DAYS

Now that I have completed all my in-patient physical therapy, the doctor has released me to go home, since I am able to take care of my needs. It was really hard to learn to do all of these things. I returned to Great Bend Hospital C.K.M.C. as an outpatient.

Getting in and out of the wheelchair was a real deal at first. I have to remember things like locking the chair so it wouldn't move and putting the pedal down. Like using the arms to help rise up out of the chair. I wasn't able to do any walking. Besides not being able to walk. I was very weak and unable to use my left arm and leg. I used a little foam ball to help build up my hand and arm. After three days of this I was able to transfer between chair and bed with help.

It was a real hard time learning to take a shower and wash my hair, even eating was a chore with just one hand. The doctors goal is to get me back to walking but I was just too weak on my left side. I had done a lot of exercises for arms and hands which I did in my wheelchair.

We did a lot of group exercises. We had a big ball we used a lot of help with coordination. After about two weeks or so of inpatient therapy I was finally ready to visit my home. This was really a good day after going over everything at home. The hospital would now make their decision. Great, they said I could go home. I got up early the next morning and got my things together and I was on my way home to stay.

I hadn't been home to stay for about three and a half weeks. In two weeks I was back at the hospital to start outpatient physical therapy,

45

one hour a day for three days a week. We started out by finding out what I could and couldn't do. We also checked muscle tone in my legs right and left.

Then the BHLE to reclaim my arm, hand and leg begins. My surgeon has already told me that I would never walk again. We started trying to see what was reasonable to be able to accomplish.

This first visit we worked on improvement in the muscle tone. Then we moved on to the arm and fingers. The second issue we got a walker out and I started to take a few short steps. The next issue was working on the weight machine for my sore legs.

As I started the next week we continued where we left off from the last week, using a walker, but making longer and longer distances. As I finished up my first month I thought I was making some real great big advances. At the close of the month I was introduced to a cane that was shaped like a little stepladder.

The cane had about an 18" square base. I started walking with the physical therapy instructor. About this time I was put on a treadmill briefly. I was also put on a weight machine briefly. Things were getting better but I still had a long way to go.

As I started my second month I was put on a program of lifting weights. I started out with 10 pound weights on both ends of the dumbbell. We worked up in weight from there. I was curling and also pressing weights. My legs were gaining strength all the time. My arm is getting stronger and my left hand is improving in grip greatly.

The third month saw many new things. I was now using a chicken foot or turkey foot cane. I was also introduced to a stairway. I had to go up eight steps and back down eight steps. You have to do this 10 times to pass this exercise.

The treadmill I will be visiting every visit for therapy. I have to do 10 minutes on it to pass the test. I have to be able to curl 30 pounds with both hands, which I can already do now. I need to be able to push up 200 pounds with my legs, but most of all I want to be able to walk with a cane.

I have now gotten to where I walked with a regular cane. I walked a half mile with the cane today, but this really wiped me out. I was so tired, all I wanted to do was sleep. I was now at a point of being dismissed from physical therapy. I have now come from a wheelchair to being able to walk in just 56 visits to a physical therapy instructor.

This seems like a real long time, but you know, that time has passed very rapidly. I have made strides, from flat on my back to being able to walk with or without a cane.

We take so many things for granted until we can't do them anymore. My walking isn't very graceful but it gets me from one place to another and that can't be all that bad. I still have a long way to go before I can walk really good. It is so good not having to go to the great Bend Hospital three days every week. I got to the point where I knew the C.K.M.C. in Great Bend very well.

We all thank God for everything He has done for us. I thank Him for being able to get around on my own two feet. God does many wondrous things that we sometimes don't deserve. We pray regularly for strength to carry on.

God really does miracles today, if you don't believe it, just look at me and where I was a year and a half ago. This tells you just what I was doing during this period of time I was taking physical therapy.

There was one thing that happened while I was an inpatient physical therapy that I am very proud of. My church choir made a trip to the Hospital C.K.M.C. and sang one Sunday afternoon in the winter for me.

Now it is time to get back to my story. It is now May 2006. I have another P.S.A. run on the 29th. It has now reached 1.100 which is too much of a jump to forget. Dr. Fesen decided to change my Taxol to a chemo called Taxatre and a second chemo was added called Crisptin. Dr. Fesen says my cancer has developed some out law cells which fight the chemo. So we aren't going to wait any longer. We are going to try something different and new and it is to work on the white spots on the bones.

This new chemo made me sick the first time, because they tried to give them to me together on the same day. There was a holiday coming up and they thought they could save time. It just didn't work. I was running on both ends. I had to go to the hospital, Clara Barton for a shot which settled my stomach.

The second time I had these two chemos I didn't get sick and everything went well, because they were not administered together. One of the new chemos takes seven hours including the pre-meds. The other chemo takes two and a half to three hours including the pre-meds.

In the month of June I have chemo on the 2, 18, and 30th. This is the three hours one. The long chemos are on the 14 and 28th, 7 to 7½ hours long. I am getting ready for the relay for life this month. The relay will be at the zoo park this year. The relay route is lit by candles which represent friends who have lost the fight with cancer. This is the route the survivors will walk.

My labs this month will be drawn at the Clara Barton Hospital on the (5, 12, 19 and 26th) of the months.

This year there were more than 50 tents and display booths set up by the city and country organizations. These groups donate to the cancer drive. They also have a number of entertainers who will come and put on a show and some will sing to the family and friends.

As the month of July is coming around the next corner my P.S.A. has now climbed to a high of 1.84 but this was as high as it will get, before falling back down to 1.010 a week later when my P.S.A. was tested again to see if the new chemo was working for me.

Now I have a new problem arising, I am starting to retain a lot of liquids in my feet and legs. I went on a pill this weekend for three days. Guess what? I took off a whopping 25 pounds and I had cramps in my legs, arms and back. I had cramps where I didn't know I had muscles. The liquid has left at least for now.

They now have me on 10 Potassium capsules a day. That is 100 megs. I am also taking 80 meg of Lasix to get rid of the water my system is retaining. My P.S.A. was run again and is now back down to .44. This is the last time it is over 0.000. Since it is under 1. I will not have a P.S.A. run for awhile.

SPECIMEN INQUIRY
HEMATOLOGY

Complete Blood Count

W.B.C.	6.3		4.8-10.8	k/mm-3
R.B.C.	4.2		8.5-5.9	m/mm-3

Hemoglobin & Hematocrit

Hemoglobin	13.7		13.5-17.5	gm/1
Hematocrit	41.3		40-52	%
M.C.V.	98		80-100	f1
M.C.H.	32.6		26-34	pg
M.C.H.C.	33.1		32-36	gm/1
R.D.W.	15.2		12-16	%
Platelet Count	224		150-350	k/mm-3
M.P.V.	7.0		7-9	f1
Neutrophils	63	H	42-62	%
Lymphocyte	25.8		20-51	%
Monocytes	6.7		1.7-9.3	%
Eosinphil	3.9		0.-7.0	%

Basophil	0.6		0.-2.0 %
Neutrophils	3.97		1.4-6.5
Lymphocyte	1.63		1.2-3.4
Monocyte	0.42		0.1-0.6
Eosinophil	0.25		0-0.7
Basophils	0.04	H	0-0.2 k/mm-3

SPECIMEN INQUIRY
CHEMISTRY

Comprehensive Metabolic Profile

Glucose	103		74-106	mg/dl
Bun	13		7-18	
Creatinine Serum	07	H	0.6-1.3	mg/dl
Bun & Creatinine Ratio	18.00		1300-2600	
Sodium	141		135-155	meg/1
Potassium	4.0		3.5-5.1	meg/1
Chloride	103		98-107	meg/1
Carbon Dioxide	30.5		21-32	mg/dl
Calcium Level	8.9		8.5-10.1	mg/dl
Total Protein	6.5		6.5-8.2	mg/dl
Albumin	3.8		3.4-5.0	gm/L
Osmolality	2.7		2.4-3.5	gm/L
Globulin	282	H	261-280	gm/L
Albumin/Globulin Ratio	1.4		1.1-2.2	
Bilirubin total	0.3		0.2-6.0	d/L

AST/SGOT	2.6	1.5-3.7	u/L
Magnesium Level	1.8	1.8-2.4	u/L
Aklaline Phosphatase	97	42-128	u/L
ALT/SGPT	49	40-65	u/L

SPECIAL CHEMISTRY

P.S.A. Diagnostic	1.840	
P.S.A. Age Dependent Ranges	49	0.1-1.4
	40-50	0.1-2.2
	50-60	0.1-3.1
	60-70	0.1-4.1
	70	0.1-4.1

JULY 2006

My Chemos this month are on the 14 and 28th. These two are the three hour chemos. My long chemos are 7½ hours and will be on the 14 and 26th of this month. My labs are drawn this month on the 3, 10, 17, 24 and 31st. On the 25th I also have a M.R.I., Cerival, Proacie and Spine.

On the 24th I have to drink Barium at bedtime. Then nothing else to eat or drink after midnight on the 25th. I have a C.T., C/A/P, M.R.I. and L. pine at the hospital C.K.M.C. I wonder if I will ever get rid of these white spots on my bones. I still believe in God's power and He will take care of me. If, it be His will, He will take this disease away from me.

AUGUST 2006

This month I am taking my chemos on the 16, and 30th. This is the 7½ hours chemo. My 3½ hours chemo I have on the 14 and 28th of this month. I see Dr. Fesen on the 2nd and 30th and his P.A. Lori. My labs for August are drawn at the Hoisington Hospital, C.B.H. on the (7, 14, 21, and 28th). As this month comes to an end my P.S.A. is now at 0.000. I will continue to take treatment for cancer as long as there is a chance these white spots could leave my bones. Here we are in the month of August and a new problem has arisen. My bladder is not draining right. I may have more problems yet, but I will cross that bridge when I come to it.

The last three days have been very high days, but you know what follows high days, you then have very low days. I know I may have pneumonia which was caused by really bad teeth. I am on a new antibiotic called Koteh for the last three days. More drugs.

SEPTEMBER 2006

We are now in the month of September. My labs this month will be drawn the 4, 11, 18 and 25th at Hoisington Hospital. My 7½ hours chemos this month will be on the 6 and 27th. My P.A., Lori, scheduled me for an (E.C.K.O.) at Hoisington Hospital at 8:30 A.M. on the 12th of this month. The (E.C.K.O.) gram is the test where they put some jelly substance on your stomach to listen to your heart. Dr. Young is my heart Doctor. He is from Wichita. He checks for congestive heart failure.

On September 22nd I had an appointment at Southwestern Urology. My new urologist is Dr. Leidick. So, now I am having a urinary track checkup. To do this procedure they put a plastic tube in the urinary track with a camera on the end of it to transmit a picture to a computer. Pictures are taken of all the inside of the urinary track also the inside of the kidneys and the bladder. This was all in good shape but my bladder isn't draining like it really should. It just doesn't drain completely. So guess what? I have another new med called Flo-Max. This med is suppose to open the bladder making it drain more completely.

I also have a sleep apnea test this week on the 29th. This test was conducted as follows: I get my pajamas together and go to the Hoisington Hospital, C.B.H. and have a P.J. party, well, not really. I go into the hospital and get ready for bed. They then put 6 or 8 probes on you and you go to sleep. While the probes transmit a signal to a computer screen for about 8 hours. Guess what? I failed the test. The next morning I went to the med-supply, Alturn-Care, and got my sleep mask. It is suppose to help by blowing air into your throat and that helps you to breath while you sleep, and scare the dog and cat away. The next day they brought me an oxygen reclainer to sleep with. What great fun. What great fun.

OCTOBER 2006

In the month of October things were very slow. Not much of anything going on. I had an appointment to see my family doctor, Dr. Nathan Knackstedt on the 5th of this month. I also see P.A. Lori on the 13 and 27th because Dr. Fesen was on his vacation in Rome Italy. Dr. Fesen told me later that he saw the Pope but I don't know, he could have been pulling my leg.

I also have an appointment at a place called, We Care at 9:30 A.M. I will be seeing a dentist called Dr. Winter to get all of my teeth pulled. I have had a hard time getting a dentist to take care of this.

My labs this month are going to be drawn at Hoisington Hospital, C.B.H. on the (2, 9, 16, 23 and 30th). I will also have a x-ray of my chest checking me out for pneumonia. I have Zometa on the same days as my chemo on the (7 and 28th). I have a yeast infection in my lungs. So now I am on antibiotics through my port on Wed., Thurs., and Fri. I will also be taking two pills a day to go along with me intravenously for the pneumonia.

This new med is called Ketek. It is very high-powered antibiotic. This med is given over 3 days. You take 3 pills the first day, then 2 pills the second day and on the 3rd day you take one pill. This is a new way to give the pills.

I also have to take Levaquin 500 mgs. This is also a new med for me. With my bad teeth I have a lot of yeast infections. They start in my mouth and go down through the body.

NOVEMBER 2006

This is a very busy month. My labs are being drawn on the 6, 13, 20, and 27th. My 7½ hours chemos are on the 8 and 22nd of the month. I also have my 3 hours chemo on the 10 and 24th. At the Heartland Cancer Center. I am still on the chemos called Crispatin for 7½ hours and Taxotre 3 to 3½ hours chemo.

I have a visit with my family doctor in Hoisington today, Dr. Nathan. This is a follow up from my x-ray last month of my lungs. I also have another visit with Dr. Liedick on the 15th of this month. Dr. Liedick is my urologist. Wanting to do what I call a peal out surgery. This is done with a laser, where they enlarge the opening leading into the bladder. I don't think I am going to have it done. Making the opening bigger will help it to drain faster but it won't make it drain anymore.

I think I have finally found a place where I can get my teeth pulled. It is a medical clinic that does a lot of work with Medicare and Medicaid patients who can't afford to go to any other place. If you are on Medicaid it is almost impossible to get any dental care. The clinic deals a lot with people who have arrived in this country for a better way of life but can't get medical help. I have called and talked to the people at Medicaid and they have approved it for me. On the 13th of this month I am scheduled at 9:30 a.m. to start getting my teeth pulled at the We Care Clinic in Great Bend Kansas. Dr. Winter thinks he will pull them in his office. We will see what happens.

The weather around here is really damp and it makes my bones ache. It is about time for the winter to start setting in again. I have to get use to it. Kansas can have some really rough winters. We haven't had any snow yet but it can't be that far down the road. Some years we go right from summer to winter but not this year.

I still haven't had much success, if any using the new sleep machine. They even said I needed a little oxygen at night. I take it off in my sleep and my wife wakes me up to tell me my mask is off and that I should put it back on my face. She tells me that I snore real bad and that is how she knows it is off in the dark. You know sometimes you can't win for losing.

I got to get the grass mowed tomorrow. I think it is suppose to be up to around 70 degrees. I am doing a lot of things right here at home. I don't take anything for granted anymore. I mow the grass with a riding mower, because I don't walk quite good enough to push a mower, but we thank God for His blessings. We continue to pray everyday and ask God to help me by getting these white spots off of my bones.

My dentist turned out to be a bit of a joke. He didn't get any of my teeth pulled. Dr. Winter worked on one wisdom tooth for two hours and didn't get it out. So, we are now back to where we started, trying to find a dentist who will cut my teeth out. It needed to be completed in a hospital setting.

Young people and children have no problem getting a dentist to take Medicaid but old people can't find dental surgeons. I guess old people don't need any dental help.

Looking back over the year we have had a lot of good times and some bad times. My wife has a couple of major surgeries. She had a rotary cup repair and a complete knee joint replacement. She is doing very well. When she had her surgery I was put in a position where I had to drive. I hadn't driven for about 2½ years. It didn't take long to get back into the swing of it.

As we look at Thanksgiving this year we have many things which we are very thankful for. The one thing is I have now lived for 2½ years with cancer in my system.

We thank God everyday for His watchful care over me. We have a lot to be thankful for. My wife and I are alive and in reasonably good health, if having cancer doesn't count. We have a really nice place to live in. A warm and dry place to sleep in the winter time and a cool place in the summer.

We had a big Thanksgiving day dinner. We had all we wanted to eat and we had many dishes of food left over for another day. We will be eating turkey for many days to come.

Tomorrow morning we are back at Clara Barton Hospital for my blood testing schedule. We all know it is up to God. We can never do anything on our own. We are only here for a short time and then we leave. We try to make the most of what ever time you and I have left on this earth.

DECEMBER 2006

In this month I have a lot of things going on. My labs will be on the (4, 11, 18, and 25th) at C.B.H. My chemos will be done on the (20 and 22nd) of this month. The chemo is on the 20th and is 7½ hours long. The 3½ hour chem is on the 22nd.

On the 12th I have a (M.R.I.) scheduled at 7:15 A.M. and a (C.T.) Scan at 10:15 for the dye and the scan was at 1:00 P.M. My (M.R.I.) was never done because I hit a deer just south of Hoisington on my way to Great Bend. That cost me about $1,500 to get my car fixed on the front end. We completed the C.T. at 10:15 A.M. and at 1:00 P.M. My M.R.I was changed to the 19thof the month. When we went out on the 19th we had a flat tire. The hospital changed the schedule still another time. This time it is for the 22nd of this month. This time the M.R.I went fine. No new white spots on my bones.

Today is Christmas Day, December 25, 2006. Christmas is a great time of the year. The weather today is very cold and extremely windy but no snow as yet but they are promising. We aren't planning on going anyplace this Christmas. My granddaughter was born on Dec. 27, eleven years ago. It is hard to have a birthday that close to Christmas. Everyone got some good thing for Christmas. We did not spend much.

It is just bout an hour before New Years. We hope this New Year will be new hope for a speedy recovery. The ball on television is starting to drop. We are counting down the last 10 seconds.

HAPPY NEW YEAR 2007
LIFE GOES ON

JANUARY 2007

January is a month with not much going on. My labs this month will continue to be drawn at C.B.H. on the 2, 8, 15, 22 and 29th of this month. I have 3 hours of chemo on the 12th. I also have 7 hours of chemo on the 31st of this month. My chemos are still Taxatre and Cripatian.

The weather is cold but it is suppose to be that way this time of year. On the15th my pastor made a visit to see me. I hadn't been to church for a couple of weeks. The weather has been so bad, we have had a lot of hard water/freezing rain. It has been below zero the last three days.

I miss church when I don't get there but I know the Lord is watching over me. I really do appreciate the people of the churches support. My family really supports me a lot.

January 21, 2007 we have about five inches of snow on the ground. It really makes it hard to get around outside with a cane. I don't have any wish to fall. Broken bones take a long time to heal.

On January 26, 2007 we are having a few nice days. The temperature today is about 50 degrees. The sun is shining very brightly on the snow. The snow is melting so fast you can almost see it leaving. I can hardly wait for it to be gone.

January 31, 2007 I am at the Heartland Center today for my 7½ hour chemo. I hope I can sleep. It makes the time go so much faster when you sleep. The pred-meds, sometimes put you to sleep for awhile. If you are tired you may sleep quite a while. The trip this morning was a little rough. We left home at 7:15 A.M. for the cancer center in Great Bend, Kansas. The ground was covered with a layer of very wet snow. The highways were very sloppy and wet.

I had a visit with Dr. Fesen today. He changed my chemo around. I now take 7½ hours of chemo and Crispatin one time every two months, and one time each month on my 3½ hour chemo Taxotre. I won't have another chemo for a month. He also raised my potassium to 12 capsules a day. When I get my potassium filled I get a whole bag full of pills. I have a lot of water retention, which flush out my potassium when I take Lasxl. I take 80 megs of Lasxl.

SPECIMEN INQUIRY
HEMATOLGOY

Complete Blood Count

W.B.C.	7.4		4.8-10.8	k/mm-3
R.B.C.	4.16	L	4.5-5.9	m/mm-3

Hemoglobin & Hematocrit

Hemoglobin	13.5		13.5-175	gm/L
Hematocrit	40.7		40.54	%
M.C.V.	98		80-100	fl
M.C.H.	32.4		26-34	pg
M.C.H.C.	33.2		32-36	g/dL
R.D.W.	15.4		12-16	%
Platelet Count	238		150-350	k/mm-3
M.P.V.	7.6		7-9	fl
Neutrophils	67.7	H	42-62	%
Lymphocyte	24.1		20-51	%
Monocyte	3.4		1.7-9.3	%
Eosinophil	4.4		0-7	%

Basophil	0.4	0-2.0 %
Neutrophils #	5.0	1.4-65
Lymphocyte #	1.80	1.2-3.4
Monocytes #	0.25	0.1-0.6
Eosinophil #	0.33	0-0.7
Basophils #	0.03	0.0.2 k/mm-3

SPECIMEN INQUIRY
CHEMISTRY

Basic Metabolic Profile

Glucose	127	74-106	mg/dL
Bun	10	7-18	mg/dL
Creatinine Serum	0.7	0.6-1.3	mg/dL
Bun & Creatinine Ratio	14.00	1300-2600	
Sodium	143	135-155	meg/L
Potassium	4.0	3.5-5.1	meg/L
Chloride	103	98-107	mmg/L
Carbon Dioxide	31.2	21-32	mg/dL
Calcium Level	8.7	8.5-10.1	mg/dL
Osmolality	286	261-280	asom/kg
Magnesium Level	1.7	1.8-2.4	mg/dL

SPECIAL CHEMISTRY

P.S.A. Diagnostic	0.0003	0.1-4.1	

P.S.A. Age Dependent
Ranges

40	0.1-1.4	MG/ML
40-50	0.1-2.0	MG/ML
50-60	0.1-3.1	MG/ML
60-70	0.1-4.1	MG/ML
70	0.1-4.4	MG/ML

FEBRUARY 2007

Today is the first day of February 2007. My blood tests will be drawn at C.B.H. on the 4, 11, 18 and 25th of the month. This is my birthday month. I was born the 10th of this month. I will be turning 68 years young. In August 2004 I would have bet I wouldn't have survived to see this birthday. I will have a short chemo on the last day of this month. I hope this is the beginning of the end of my chemo, but I will leave it up to God to take care of it.

The 2nd of February we have a snowstorm coming in. I have changed my chemo to the 1st on Thursday at 10:00 A.M. at the cancer center. I don't have to see Dr. Fesen this week so it really works out great.

February 7, 2007, my wife's birthday. We celebrate both of our birthdays the same week, the same days. A few days before my birthday I started to get a lot of cards. I don't usually get more than a few cards. This year was different. My wife finally told me, she had a card shower for me. So far I have gotten a total of 28 cards. It must be working.

I got several nice things, but just what do you get for an old grandpa. Life has been good so far this year. My cancer seems to be improving. I am beginning to think that maybe I can see the light at the end of the tunnel. I still have a ways to go yet.

The weather is bad, we have about 6 or 7" of snow on the ground. It is very wet and cold. The temperature is 15 degrees with a 25 mile an hour wind. Making the wind chill of 18 degrees below zero. At 18 degrees below zero the wind chill can really freeze you.

Today is February 24, 2007 the weather is really beautiful. The temperature is about 50 degrees. You can really see the snow melting. Here in Kansas if you don't like the weather just wait a few minutes and it will change. In Kansas the wind blows everyday one way or the other.

We had a good day at church. I am thankful to my God that I am able to go to church. I put my trust in Him that He will take care of me.

I have an appointment to see Dr. Fesen's P.A. (physicians assistant), Lori at 10:30 A.M. on the 30th at which time I get another Neulast short. This shot is given to help with bone pain and energy. Energy is something that cancer seems to rob you of.

I have a M.R.I Lumber Sack test at C.K.M.C. Central Kansas Medical Center in Great Bend, Kansas. I also have two new medications. One is called Amoxicillan, an antibiotic. The other drug is called Bezoative, a decongestant for my hacky cough. Dr. Nathan thought maybe I was coming down with pneumonia.

MARCH 2007

We have a major storm coming in tonight. We are now under a tornado watch. The tornado sirens are now going off. We are not under a tornado warning. If it rains very hard tonight we will have problems getting into Great Bend tomorrow. Water crosses the highway that laves out of town to the south. The all clear has sounded so we are out of the wood again.

I took my granddaughter to school this morning. She usually rides the bus but I was up early this morning. I wake up around 5:00 in the morning. Everyone else likes to get up much later. We continue to pray for healing from God as we continue to fight this dreaded disease.

We are suppose to have real nice weather most all of this week. It is a great time of the year. When winter turns to spring. The birds come north and all the pretty flowers start blooming. It is time to plant our garden with anticipation of the fresh vegetables. Jesus must have really like green, because he made so many things green. Almost all vegetation on the planet is green.

SPECIMEN INQUIRY
HEMATOLOGY

Complete Blood Count

W.B.C.	7.1		4.8-10.8	k/mm-3
R.B.C.	4.41	L	4.5-5.9	m/mm-3

Hemoglobin & Hematocrit

Hemoglobin	14.2		13.5-17.5	gm/dL
Hematocrit	43.3		40-54	%
M.C.V.	98		80-100	F1
M.C.H.	32.2		26-34	Pd
M.C.H.C.	32.8		32-36	gm/dL
R.D.W.	15.6		12-16	%
Platelet Count	254		150-360	k/mm-3
M.P.V.	7.3		7-9	f1
Neutrophils	67.8	H	42-62	%
Lymphocyte	22.9		20-51	%
Monocytes	5.5		1.7-9.3	%
Eosinophil	9.3		0-7	%

Basophil	05	0-2.0 %
Neutrophils #	4.82	1-4-6.5
Lymphocyte #	1.63	1.2-3.4
Monocyte #	0.39	0.1-0.6
Eosinophil #	.023	0-0.7
Basophil #	0.04	0-0.2 K/mm-3

SPECIMEN INQUIRY
CHEMISTRY

Basic Metabolic Profile

Basic Metabolic Profile

Glucose	114		74-105	mg/d1
Bun	14		7-8	mg/d1
Creatinine Serum	0.8		0.6-1.3	mg/d1
Bun & Creatinine Ratio	20.00		6.00-2600	
Sodium	141		135-155	meg/L
Potassium	4.0		3.5-5.1	meg/L
Chloride	102		98-107	meg/L
Carbon Dioxide	33.8	H	21-32	mmol/L
Calcium Level	96		8.5-10.1	mg/L
Osmolality	283	H	261-280	uosm/kg
Magnesium Level	2.0		1.8-2.4	mg/dL

SPECIAL CHEMISTRY

P.S.A. Diagnostic	0.006	0.1-4.1

Age P.S.A. Dependency
Ranges

Age	P.S.A. Range	
40	0.1-1.4	mg/m1
40-50	0.1-2.0	mg/m1
50-60	0.1-3.1	mg/m1
60-70	0.1-4.1	mg/m1
70	0.1-4.4	mg/m1

APRIL 2007

April came in like a lamb very mild and pleasant, but it didn't really last very long. As the first week came along. We are now expecting a late winter snowstorm. This year is really becoming a very strange year for unusual weather patterns. We had a lot of spring storms already and it is only April.

April is a real pretty month. I got a tractor out and mowed the grass. I am going to plant some roses tomorrow. The air is so fresh today. The birds are singing and all of nature starts anew. I bought some garden plants and tomatoes. We talk a lot about the weather but if we were controlling the weather, just think how bad it would be with some wanting rain and others don't want it. Lets just leave it like it is, okay!

My labs are being drawn on the 2, 9, 16, 23 and 20th. I have just one chemo this month. On the 23rd. It is a 3 hours chemo called Taxotre at the Heartland Cancer Center in Great Bend Kansas. I also had 20 met and Neulasta on the 27th of this month.

On the 16th of this month I had a visit with Dr. Arnold to have a surgery scheduled for the removal of a mole from my back. Since I have cancer they don't want to wait around on moles. On the 20th I had the small mole removed. The mole was a fibrous growth and it was not cancerous. Dr. Arnold did my surgery and it only took about 30 minutes or so.

I am scheduled to see Dr. Fesen's physicians assistant, Lori on the 27th of this month. I always enjoy seeing her. She is such a good person. We had a Friday the 13th appointment. I have always said that 13 was my lucky number.

Dr. Fesen has also taken me off of a cancer med called Casidex. So far my P.S.A. has stayed at 0.000 and it has been that way for an entire year now. This sounds really great too. The P.S.A. is my cancer indicator of my cancer growth.

MAY 2007

The month of May is such a pretty time of the year. The life is returning to the trees and the grass is getting green. We have our vegetables planted and we wait for the seeds to sprout and put forth a crop.

Today is the first of May. My P.S.A. is still at 0.000 which is really very good news. I started my regiment of blood tests. This month my labs will be drawn on the 7, 14, 21 and 28th. At the hospital in Hoisington, Kansas C.B.H. I have to see Dr. Fesen on May 2nd for a checkup. There will not be a P.S.A. drawn this month. I have Zomet and Neulasta twice this month. I have my chemo on the 23rd on the 4th Wednesday of this month. This chemo is the 7½ hour variety which is Crispatine. I will receive Zometa and a Neulasta shot on the 30th at 11:00 A.M. Dr. Fesen says I am doing very well.

I have a C.T. scan of my sinuses at 10:00 A.M. on the 10th at C.K.M.C. in Great Bend, Kansas. They are checking my sinuses for a blockage. I will be seeing Dr. Fesen's P.A., Lori, at 11:15 A.M. on the 25th of May. My C.T. scan came back clear no blockage, but of course I already knew that.

As the month of May becomes a thing of the past, we will fill out more paperwork. So far we haven't had any solid source of help in getting my paperwork done and still no help with my teeth.

Next month will be the relay for life. This year it will be at the college Northeast of Great Bend. The weather has been so we that they moved it to the college (Barton Community College) just north of Great Bend, Kansas.

We go to church each week and it is good to be able to be walking in the front door. I continue to have very good support from my church family and also my home family.

JUNE 2007

Today we welcome the month of June. My labs this month are being drawn on the 4, 11, 18 and 25th. My labs this month are C.B.C., C.M.P., B.M.P. and of course the P.S.A. I have a M.R.I. at 7:30 A.M. at C.K.M.C. Central Medical Center in Great Bend, Kansas. My tests were real good. Showing improvement over the last ones.

I see Dr. Fesen on the 13th of this month at 2:45 P.M. A quick check of my lungs and my heart and I am on my way. I will also see the P.A. at 10:30 A.M. at the Cancer Center for more checkups on the 22nd. I have 3 hours of chemo and Zometa on the 27th of this month. I also have a shot of Neulasta on the 27th. I sometimes wonder how they can keep pumping these liquids in but never having to take anything out. This may really sound strange, but when you have a lot of time to think, well, you know what I mean.

Today is the first of June, the sixth month of this year. The cancer relay is scheduled on the 8th of this month at the Barton County Community College B.C.C.C. the relay went off very well. There was a large crowd of survivors and their families and friends. The country sponsors had a lot of display tens, food, drinks and novelties. The parade and music went on most of the night.

I hope my bones are getting better. We are trying to get rid of the white spots on my bones. All my M.R.I. and C.T. are checking these white spots. We continue to pray for Gods healing.

On June 13, 2007, when I saw Dr. Fesen I was surprised to see him upset the apple cart on my chemos. He took my 7½ hour chemo away. Then he took my 3½ hour chemo Taxitire away. In their place he put a chemo I took about 2½ year ago. Taxol was one of the first chemos I ever took in the beginning. My P.S.A. is now at 0.000. I will now take Taxol twice a month or every 2 weeks.

This means about 5 hours of chemo a month. This should help with water retention. That will lower my Lasix and then my water retention goes down which will lower my potassium capsule intake. Right now I take 12 capsules a day and 80 mg of Lasix, a water diuretic.

While I was on Crispatin I started gaining weight. I had lost 60 pounds before I had my surgery. This chemo has caused me to gain back all the weight I had lost before I had surgery and more. This is getting to be a real problem. It is not hard to put on weight but taking it off is still another story. Some people stay so think but not me. Other people lose weight and I always find it.

I get to go to church every week and that can't be all too bad. Everything is not a bowl of cherries, but it is better than being a bowl of lemons.

We sometimes think something just can't happen to us. It just doesn't pay to be too boisterous about these things, and of course, how we eat has a lot to do with this disease. God will heal us if it be His will. Sometimes we don't understand why God does some things but His will be done. in His own time and way.

JULY 2007

July has now arrived in Kansas, along with its heat, but this year is a little different because we have rain along with the heat. It seems like it rains three or four times every month. The tomatoes are doing well and the flowers are blooming. Everything is in bloom. The grass stayed green all summer long. I have to mow every week. The farmers market is loaded with many vegetables and fruits. It has been too hot for my flowers. The roses have all died. Maybe my thumb is brown now instead of green.

In the month of July I have my labs drawn on 2; 9, 16, 23 and 30th. My chemo is on the 11 and 25th. I think I am coming along very well. I have Neulasta on the 11th and Zometa and Neulasta on the 25th of this month. I haven't gotten sick on chemo and that is a real good thing. I have watched many people get sick as a dog. I also had an extra blood test on the 25th to check my Vitamin D Level.

I had my back checked today by Dr. Arnold, and has released me. No more checkups for my back. I saw Dr. Fesen on the 11th just before having my chemo. My P.S.A. is continuing to stay put at 0.000. Almost all of my blood tests were good, only three were off a little. The white count is always off a little.

SPECIMEN INQUIRY
HEMATOLOGY

Complete Blood Count

W.B.C.	10.7		4.8-10.8	k/mm-3
R.B.C.	4.231	L	4.5-5.9	m/mm-3

Hemoglobin & Hematocrit

Hemoglobin	14.0		13.5-17.5	gm/L
Hematocrit	42.5		40-54	%
M.C.V.	99		80-100	fl
M.C.H.	32.5		26-34	pg
M.C.H.C.	32.9		32-36	g/dL
R.D.W.	15.4		12-16	%
Platelet Count	293		150-350	k/mm-3
Neutrophils	75	H	42-62	%
Lymphocyte	19.3	L	20-51	%
Monocytes	3.1		1.7-9.3	%
Eosinophil	2.2		0.7	%
Basophil	0.2		0-2.0	%

Neutrophils #	8.05	H	1.4-6.5
Lymphocyte #	2.09		1.2-3.4
Monocyte #	0.33		0.1-0.6
Eosinophil #	0.24		0-0.7
Basophils #	0.02		0-0.1 k/mm-3
M.P.V.	7.2		7-9 fl

SPECIMENT INQUIRY
CHEMISTRY

Basic Metabolic Profile

Glucose	101		74-106	mg/dL
Bun	11		7-18	mg/dL
Creatinine Serum	0.8	H	0.6-1.3	mg/dL
Bun & Creatineine Ratio	13.00		6.00-2600	meg/L
Sodium	144		135-155	meg/L
Potassium	3.7		3.5-5.1	meg/L
Chloride	104		98-104	meg/L
Carbon Dioxide	29.7		21-32	mmol/L
Calcium Level	9.0		8.5-10.1	mg/dL
Osmolality	286	H	261-280	uosm/kg
Magnesium Level	1.6	L	1.8-2.4	mg/dL

McKESSON
Empowering Healthcare

Name: **Deitsch Jr, Lloyd**
DOB: **10-Feb-1939**
ID: **033029**
Study Date: **11-Dec-2006**

MRI OF THE LUMBAR SPINE WITH AND WITHOUT CONTRAST, 12/11/06

Comparison is made with the prior study dated 07/31-06.

The lumbar vertebral bodies are well-aligned. Vertebral body heights are well maintained. There is a somewhat mottled appearance to the lumbar vertebral bodies that may be on the basis of osteoporosis. This is somewhat similar to the prior examination. This may be related to diffuse metastases, and is unchanged. The lumbar vertebral bodies are well-aligned. Vertebral body heights are well maintained. No definite evidence for acute compression fracture is identified. There is neural foraminal narrowing, particularly at L4-5 bilaterally, and mildly at L6-S1.

Axial images obtained at L1-2 shows minimal disc bulge.

At L2-3 mild disc bulge flattens the anterior thecal sac, and is similar to prior examination.

At L3-4 mild disc bulge also flattens the anterior thecal sac, contributing to mild spinal canal narrowing. Mild spinal canal narrowing is also seen at L2-3. This is unchanged since prior exam.

At L4-5 circumferential disc bulge and left ventricular hypertrophy contribute to moderate spinal canal stenosis. Lateral disc bulge contributes to bilateral neural foraminal narrowing, which may affect the L4 nerve root.

At L5-S1 there is mild disc bulge with convex mass effect on the anterior thecal sac.

Subcutaneous edema is seen in the subcutaneous tissues posteriorly, particularly at the level of L1 and L2.

IMPRESSION:
1. There is a mottled appearance to the lumbar sacral vertebral bodies, which may represent diffuse metastases which are unchanged.
2. There is again noted moderate spinal canal stenosis at L4-5 and circumferential disc bulge with ligamentum flavum hypertrophy and bilateral neural foraminal narrowing. This is unchanged since prior examination.
3. Mild disc bulges at L2-3 and L3-4 are again noted, contributing to mild spinal canal narrowing.
4. Circumferential disc bulge at L5-S1 contributes to bilateral neural foraminal narrowing, and is also unchanged.
5. Essentially no significant change since prior examination.

Dictated By: CABRERA,ARNOLD R MD 12/20/2006 0832
Released By: (Electronic Signature) SIGNED
WILSON,GARY L DO 12/20/2006 1614
Transcribed: ETR 12/20/2006 1014

Signed by: Signed at:

On the Monday, July 30th I have another bone scan. I continue to have these bone scans to check on the white spots on my bones. I think I keep C.K.M.C. in business. I hope to get off of chemo real soon. I also have Zometa to help me with my bone pain. I don't have another P.S.A. run until next month. Dr. Fesen is really taking good care of me.

AUGUST 2007

This month comes around with a lot of blistering heat, 100 plus and a lot more rain than we usually get in the month of August. This month has been a very lack luster month. Really not much going on with my cancer anyway.

I have my labs drawn on the (6, 13, 20 and 27th). All my labs will be drawn at the hospital in Hoisington, Kansas C.B.H. Clara Barton Hospital. The one good thing in this month is I am starting to loose some of this weight. I have packed it on since I started this chemo called Crispatin. The 7 hour chemo I was taking a few months ago.

I have an appointment to see Dr. Fesen on the 8th at 9:15 A.M. I have my 3 hours of chemo Taxol and my shot of Neulasta. My other chemo will be on the 22nd. I have Zometa and Neulasta with my chemo this time. I haven't had a M.R.I. for a few months now. I am sure one is in the making sooner or later.

Three years ago this month I was diagnosed with cancer. I was down in bed almost completely paralyzed on one side. Unable to walk or use my left arm and leg. Today I can walk and use my left arm, hand and my leg. What a blessing this has turned out to be. I thank God that my life was been spared.

My P.S.A. has remained at 0.000 for many months, which is very good. I got a copy of my labs again today. I don't know what everything on the Specimen Inquiry/lab report means, but i have learned a lot over the years about what my meds and lab reports say.

I have gone through four different kinds of chemos. I don't know how many different kinds of antibiotics I have taken and the pre-meds I have no idea about them. I just leave it up to Dr. Fesen and Dr. Nathan. I have a lot of confidence in them and in their staff of regular nurses at the Heartland Cancer Center in Great Bend, Kansas.

God has played a very large part in my lab reports. We pray daily for help but we don't forget to thank Him for His blessings. We spend a lot of time at the hospital here in Hoisington C.B.H. When I go in everyone knows me by my first name. They say when everyone knows you, you have been there way to often.

Going every Monday for labs can get to be a real nuisance but we continue to have blood drawn at C.B.H. Clara Barton Hospital every Monday. All my M.R.I., C.T., and bone scans are done at C.K.M.C. Central Kansas Medical Center located in Great Bend, Kansas.

I have had more than 300 shots and more than 350 blood tests and as of yet I haven't come down with any infections. My port has been in now more than three years and it is still working. I must be doing something right.

I have included my lab reports to show how much they have changed from time to time. I can remember having 8 to 10 markers. So things are improving nicely. I couldn't have done it on my own.

The weather continues to cool down now. We have had temperatures that were almost record breaking for the end of this month. You know Kansas, the weather is something we can't do anything about but talk about it.

SEPTEMBER 2007

We enter into the ninth month of the year. Three more months and we will begin the new year of 2008. We don't want to rush things. I would like to be greatly improved by the end of the year.

The labs this month are on 3, 10, 17 and 24th. I have a P.S.A. lab on the 17th of this month. All my labs are drawn at the hospital in Hoisington C.B.H. Clara Barton Hospital. The majority of my labs have been done at C.B.H.

My chemos this month are on the 5th and 19th. My 3 hour chemo and Neulasts shot are on the 5th. On the 19th I have the 3 hours of chem, my Neulasta shot and Zometa. To top it off there is an appointment on the 19th to see Dr. Fesen. I hope he is in a good mood like he was last month.

I slept through half of my chemo today. I got a copy of my labs. I don't know what I am doing but I must be doing it right. I got done today just before 12:00 noon. I had good new. I lost 6 pounds. You aren't suppose to gain weight while you are on chemo but I gained a bunch while I was on the two chemos Cripatin and Taxatire.

My P.S.A. continued to stay down at 0.000. It has been 1½ years since my P.S.A. was anything but 0.000. We hope and pray that it will stay down. The P.S.A. is a cancer indicator of my system showing any growth. I will continue to try to get the spot off my bones.

Dr. Fesen is really happy with my progress so far. I still have a long way to go but I will be working on these spots until they are all gone and I am cancer free. I guess I did something wrong because my labs aren't very good this month.

OCTOBER 2007

The next P.S.A. will be run on the 4th week in October. The month of October is upon us now. The weather today is very hot. I have my first chemo of this month on the third. My other chemos are on the 3, 17 and 31st. Three chemos this month.

My labs are drawn on the 1, 8, 15, 22 and 29th. All labs are C.B.C., C.M.P. and MG except for C.B.C., P.S.A., C.M.P. and MG will be done on the 29th. I will continue doing 3 chemos which aren't too bad. I continue to take chemo and I don't get sick.

The weather has finally turned cool. The temperature is a mild 48 degrees this morning. I now have an infection in my lungs and they put me on a z-pack and a shot in my bottom. That was great fun don't you know. This antibiotic is called Azithromycin, 250 mgs, another antibiotic to add to my collection.

I went to the cancer center today. My cold and sore throat doesn't seem to be getting any better. I saw the physicians assistant, Lori, which didn't really help very much. She told me to continue to take the z pack. She answered several of my questions that I had, also my weight was down a couple of more pounds.

On the Wednesday the 3rd of this month I went to the Heartland Cancer Center to have chemo. I found out my magnesium level was very low so I had one bag of magnesium and a bag of Zometa for my bones. My bones were really starting to ache. It take me 3½ hours to have all of this done. My labs were also much better today than the last time. Praise God. My next chemo and a visit with Dr. Fesen was on the 31st of this month. I also had a shot of Neulasta on the 31st.

We are under a major storm watch until midnight. This time of year you can't be sure of the type of storm. It could be a thunderstorm or a tornado, or even an early ice storm. I hope we don't get any hard water, you know hail. Well I have to go for now.

The next day. The weather turned cold. We may even get our first frost this week, but actually it is a little early. If it frosts there goes all of our planets. It is time that we begin closing out the month of October 2007 in a few days.

SPECIMEN INQUIRY
HEMATOLOGY

Complete Blood Count

W.B.C.	12.6	H	4.8-10.8	k/mm-3
R.B.C.	4.52		4.5-5.9	m/mm-3

Hemoglobin & Hematocrit

Hemoglobin	14.8		13.5-17.5	gm/L
Hematocrit	44.4		40-54	%
M.C.V.	98.0		80-100	gm/L
M.C.H.	32.7		26-34	fl
M.C.H.C.	33.3		32-36	pd
R.D.W.	14.5		12-16	%
Platelet Count	219		150-350	k/mm-3
M.P.V	7.6		7-9	fl
Neutrophils	65.2	H	42-62	%
Lymphocyte	22.7		20-51	%
Monocytes	9.4	H	1.7-9.3	%
Eosinophil	2.2		0.-7	%

Basophil	0.5		0.-2.0	%
Neutrophils #	8.21	H	1.4-6.5	
Lymphocyte #	2.86		1.2-3.4	
Monocytes #	1.18	H	0.1-0.6	
Eosinophil #	0.28		0-0.7	
Basophils #	0.06		0-0.6	k/mm-3

Baseball and the World Series are over and won by Boston. High school football, college and pro-football are getting started and it won't be long till track, field and volleyball will be done also. The rodeo and nextre racing will be finished. When you aren't very active seasons come and go in a fairly slow manner, but time seems to flash by with all of the activity of my hospital and doctor visits.

All of the outdoor sports are about finished. The weather is all messed up again. Wouldn't you just know it. We haven't had any snow yet, but there is always tomorrow. We have had several freezes and one that was hard on the tomatoes and flowers. They are all dried up.

Today is October 31, 2007. I have my chemo today at the Heartland Cancer Center in Great Bend, Kansas. I had to see Dr. Fesen for a checkup today. I had 2½ hours of Taxol and mg. I also had a Neulasts shot. My P.S.A. was still at 0.000. On my last lab report everything seems to be coming along very well. I would still like to be off chemo by the first of the New Year.

MANUAL DIFFERENTAL	N/C			
Neutrophil	4.40		34-62	%
Band	40.0	H	0-5	%
Lymphocy	3.0		25-33	%
Monocytes	1.18	H	0.1-06	
Eosinophil	0.28		0-07	
Basophil	0.06		0-06	k/mm-3

MANUAL DIFFERENTAL	N/C			
Neutrophils #	44.0		54-62	%
Band #	30.0	H	0-5	%
Lymphocyte #	17.0	L	25-33	%
Monocytes #	4.0		3-7	%
Eosinophil #	4.0		1-3	%

SPECIMEN INQUIRY
CHEMISTRY

Basic Metabolic Profile

Glucose	120		74-106	wmo/L
Bun	12		7-18	mg/dL
Creatinine Serum	.09		0.6-1.3	mg/dL
Bun & Creatinine Ratio	13.00		600-2600	
Sodium	141		135-155	meg/L
Potassium	4.2		3.5-5.1	meg/L
Chloride	102		98-107	meg/L
Carbon Dioxide	28.9		21-32	mm-3/L
Calcium Level	9.3		8.5-10.1	mg/dL
Osmolality	282	H	261-280	usoh/L
Magnesium Level	1.7	L	1.8-2.4	mg/L

SPECIAL CHEMISTRY

P.S.A. Diagnostic	0.000	0.1-4.1
	40	0.1-1.4

40-50	0.1-2.0
50-60	0.1-3.1
60-70	0.1-4.1
70	0.1-4.4

NOVEMBER 2007

This month my labs are being drawn on the 5, 12, 19 and 26th. The labs to be drawn are C.B.C., B.M.P. and mg, except on the 26th which will also have a P.S.A. All my labs this month will be drawn at C.B.H. Clara Barton Hospital in Hoisington, Kansas.

My chemos this month are on the 14 and 28th. On the 14th I have chemo Taxol, Zometa and a shot of Neulasta. This all took about 3½ hours. On Friday I will be seeing Dr. Fesen's physical therapist/Lori at 9:45 A.M. at the Cancer Center.

The Zometa will help my bone pain. It has now been three full years since I started chemo. It just seems like it hasn't been that long. But at times it seems to past very fast.

The weather is cold and windy. The temperature is about 25 degrees this morning. This is a major freeze, ice everywhere. It is very hard to drive against 20 mile per hour winds. But we still don't have any show. Tomorrow I will be seeing Dr. Fesen's P.A., Lori. Dr. Fesen is on vacation again. I don't know where he has gone this time. The last time he went to Rome, Italy.

I have my appointment with physicians assistant, Lori. She cleared up a lot of questions I was having about my chemo. My chemo will be used for now at least as a maintenance drug. I now have an appointment with another new doctor by the name of Dr. Garcia.

Dr. Garcia specializes in the sinus field. They still think that my sinuses are causing some of my stuffed up head and congestion. I enjoy seeing the physicians assistant, Lori. She is such a friendly person and so full of life. My appointment is on Tuesday, January 8th, 2008.

I saw my family doctor yesterday. Dr. Nathan examined me and said my sugar is a little elevated, so I have a new drug called Byetta. Byetta is used for blood sugar control and also for weight control. I should lose between 3 and 5 pounds a month. It doesn't seem like very much but every little bit helps. I go back and see him in a month.

SPECIMEN INQUIRY
HEMATOLOGY

Complete Blood Count

W.B.C.	7.0		4.8-10.8	k/mm-3
R.B.C.	4.2	L	4-5-5.9	m/mm-3

Hemoglobin & Hematocrit

Hemoglobin	13.4	L	13.5-17.5	gm/L
Hematocrit	41.1		50-54	%
M.C.V.	98.0		80-100	fl
M.C.H.	32.0		26-34	g/dl
M.C.H.C.	34.0		32-36	g/dl
R.D.W.	15.3		12-16	%
Platelet Count	245		150-350	k/mm-3
M.P.V.	7.0		7-9	fl
Neutrophils	64.7	H	42-62	%
Lymphocyte	27.9		20-51	%
Monocytes	3.2		1.7-9.3	%
Eosinophil	3.8		0-7	%

Basophil	0.4	H	0.-2.0	%
Neutrophils #	4.53		1.4-6.5	
Lymphocyte #	1.95		1.2-3.4	
Monocytes #	0.22		0.1-0.6	
Eosinophil #	0.27		0-0.7	k/mm-3
Basophils #	0.03		0.-0.2	k/mm-3

SPECIMEN INQUIRY
CHEMISTRY

Basic Metabolic Profile

Glucose	9.2		74-106 mg/dL
Bun	14		7-18 mg/dL
Creatinine Serum	.09	H	0.6-1.3 mg/dL
Bun & Creatinine Ratio	15.00		6.00-2600
Sodium	140		135-155 meg/L
Potassium	3.6		3.5-5.1 meg/L
Chloride	10.0		98-107 meg/L
Carbon Dioxide	29.7		21-32 mmol/L
Calcium Level	9.1		8.5-10.1 mg/dL
Osmolality	280		261-280 uosa/L
Magnesium Level	1.7		1.8-2.4 mg/dL

SPECIAL CHEMISTRY

P.S.A. Diagnostic	0.000	0.1-4.1
P.S.A. Age Dependent Ranges	40	0.1-1.4

Ages (Years)	40-50	0.1-2.0
	50-60	0.1-3.1
	60-70	0.1-4.1
	70	0.1-4.4

Thanksgiving is coming very fast. We will be staying home this year. This time of year is for family and friends to get together and enjoy a good meal and be thankful for being alive. As we relive this year we have many things we are very thankful for. Well, got to go for now.

A new problem has arisen as I seem to be coming back to my old self. I am having trouble sleeping at night. I wake up at a time between 1:30 and 3:00 in the morning and can't get back to sleep. It is a bad time and you don't want to wake someone up to talk to them.

I sometimes get a little depressed, but I listen to my music and read the Bible to help me relax and to back to sleep. I have a lot of music, C.D.'s and cassettes. I also have the Bible on a C.D. My walkman C.D. player is my best friend at night. I like to watch the daylight approach into a new day.

Thanksgiving Day is here. We are busy, busy all day long. We are having a real good meal. This year we are having turkey, mash potatoes, dressing, noodles, cranberry sauce, sweet potatoes, corn, beans, pie (apple and pumpkin) and two kinds of cake and many more dishes. Everyone has a lot to be thankful for this year.

My daughter has recovered from her accident last May and is back on her E.M.T. job working on the Ambulance here in Hoisington, Kansas. My wife is doing very well with her knee replacement. Me, I am doing pretty well. If in fact you can be doing very well while taking chemo for cancer treatment.

O, yes! It has finally snowed. About noon on Thanksgiving Day it started with a few flurries. By the time evening had come we had 2 inches on the ground. On Friday it continued to snow lightly.

Today is Monday, November 26, 2007 and we have snow on the ground. They say it is suppose to get up to 45 degrees, bye bye snow. I hope. I go to the Hoisington Hospital C.B.H. in Kansas.

I went to the hospital for my regular blood test. I have a P.S.A. scheduled this week. I hope it continues to come out at 0.000. Next Wednesday on the 28th I have another round of chemo, but I don't see the doctor this week.

I had my round of chemo and a Neulasta shot. Everything went off like clockwork, like on time. I arrived early at about 8:45 A.M. at the cancer center. I got hooked up at 9:15 which was about 15 minutes early for pre-meds and then my Taxol. Everything took about 2 hours and 45 minutes, as I was finished at 12:00 P.M.

I got a copy of my labs today. My P.S.A. was at 0.000 again. This is where we wanted it to stay at. This basically means I don't have any active cancer cells growing in my system. I have had no readings over 0.000 for nearly a year.

The weather has made a big change again today. It is about 60 degrees this afternoon. The weather plays a big role in how you feel. Tomorrow they are talking about another big change. In Kansas they say (if you don't like the weather, wait a little while and it will change).

Next week I have blood work at C.B.A. and some more scans at C.K.M.C. (Central Kansas Medical Center) in Great Bend, Kansas. I got my Barium today and it must be taken tonight before I go to bed. No more food to eat and nothing to drink after midnight. In the morning I will receive another 6 ounces of Barium to drink and nothing else till after my scans.

I am hoping and praying the white spots on my bones will be gone. When my prostrate cancer metastasized and moved up the spinal column, it left a lot of white spots on my bones, which, if left untreated can become active and spread further throughout my skeletal system.

So we continue to take chemo treatments and also Neulasta shots. Hoping these treatments will cause these spots to leave. I pray regularly for healing of my system. God can do anything and we trust that He will intervene and heal me, and all of these white spots will suddenly be gone. We continue to have M.R.I and scans to keep everything in check.

SPECIMEN INQUIRY
HEMATOLOGY

Complete Blood Count

W.C.B.	7.9		4.8-10.8	k/mm-3
R.B.C.	4.2	L	4.5-5.9	m/mm-3

Hemoglobin & Hematocrit

Hemoglobin	13.8		13.5-17.5	gm/L
Hematocrit	4.14		40-54	%
M.C.V.	97		80-100	fl
M.C.H.	32.5		26-34	pg
M.C.H.C.	33.4		32-36	g/dl
R.D.W.	15.1		12-16	%
Platelet Count	248		150-350	k/mm-3
M.P.V.	7.0		7-9	fl
Neutrophils	69.2	H	42-62	%
Lymphocyte	33.9		20-51	%
Monocytes	3.8		1.7-9.3	%
Eosinophil	2.6		0-7	%

Basophil	0.5	0-2.0	%
Neutrophils #	5.49	1.4-6.5	
Lymphocyte #	1.90	1.20-3.4	
Monocyte #	0.30	0.1-0.6	
Eosinophil #	0.21	0-0.7	
Basophils #	0.04	0-0.2	k/mm-3

SPECIMEN INQUIRY
CHEMISTRY

Basic Metabolic Profile

Glucose	92		74-106	mg/dL
Bun	14		7-18	mg/dL
Creatinine Serum	.09	H	0.6-1.3	mg/dL
Bun & Creatinine Ratio	15.00		6.00-2600	
Sodium	140		135-155	meg/L
Potassium	3.6		3.5-5.1	meg/L
Carbon Dioxide	29.7		21-32	mo1/L
Calcium Level	9.1		8.5-10.1	mg/dL
Osmolality	280		261-280	ussm/kg
Magnesium Level	1.7		1.8-2.4	mg/dL

SPECIAL CHEMISTRY

P.S.A. Diagnostic	0.000	0.1-4.1	mg/L
Age Range	40	0.1-1.4	
	40-50	0.1-2.0	

97

50-60	0.1-3.1
60-70	0.1-4.1
70	0.1-4.4

DECEMBER 2007

Today is the first day of December 2007. The weather is terrible. We are forecast to have some freezing rain changing to snow tonight. It is getting colder all the time. Sunday morning no snow or ice, just rain. It looks like we beat the bullet one more time.

Monday, December 3, 2007. I went to the hospital in Hoisington, C.B.H. to have regular blood test drawn. They were very busy this morning. I had to wait an hour for my turn in the lab. My lab tests today are C.B.C., B.M.P. and mg and I also had a flu shot.

Today Wednesday December 5th. I have an appointment at C.K.M.C. at 9:15 A.M. for a C.T. scan which means I drank 10 ounces of Barium last night and will get another 6 ounces before starting my C.T. scan.

When I had a bone scan last month. They put me on a moving table that moves in and out through a donut shaped laser scanner. After they scan you one time, they pull you out and put a shunt in the back of your hand and inject dye in your vein. Wait 15 minutes and put you back in the scanner where the dye will glow white in the scanner.

I think today I could have made light bulbs burn. Everything went very well. My next chemo is next week on December 12, 2007. I also see Dr. Fesen before having my chemo.

Today is Monday December 10th. I am at the Hoisington Hospital C.B.H. for my weekly blood to be drawn, C.M.P., B.M.P. and Mg. It is really a nice day, but tonight a major ice storm is scheduled to move into the state. It started raining and freezing Monday night and continued most of the day and evening on Tuesday.

The cancer center called me today, Tuesday and cancelled my appointment because of the bad weather. Tree limbs were down and heavy ice covered everything.

They rescheduled my appointment from Wednesday 12th to Friday the 14th at 9:15 A.M. at the Heartland Cancer Center. The next time I see Dr. Fesen is on Wednesday the 19th of December. Maybe the ice will be gone by then. I also have an appointment to see Dr. Nathan on December 18th at 10:00 in the morning.

Today is Friday December 14th. I went to the Heartland Cancer Center in Great Bend, Kansas today. When I got there at 8:30 A.M.

there was only three patients in the center. One hour later there was 40 patients and by the time it was noon, there were 60 patients.

I got started really early today and I was finished at about noon. The same nurse administered my chemo today. She always does a real good job. Everything went very well. My port has worked without any trouble for nearly four years now. I have known people who had trouble in the first two or tree months.

I had a 1½ hours chemo, 45 minutes of pre-meds and ½ hour of Zometa for a total of about 3 hours and a Neulasta shot. I was done by noon. This day was an average cloudy, and dull looking day. The noon temperature was a balmy 24 degrees.

My wife and I met our daughter at noon for lunch, at the Pizza Hut. While we were eating it started to snow. When we came out it had already snowed an inch or two. It was coming down at an inch an hour. The visual driving distance was ½ mile ahead. They are predicting 7 to 10 inches and ending sometime tomorrow.

We will miss church tomorrow again but God has kept us safe through the storms and now we have another one. We put our lives in Gods hands and He will protect us from harm.

Today I went to the hospital for my blood test, in the problems of cancellations because of the two storms. My doctor or the Cancer Center had failed to send new orders to the hospital in Hoisington C.B.H., but after a few calls were made they faxed new orders. My blood tests were drawn and I was on my way home.

The temperature this morning is just one degree above zero. Burr Burr. The car moaned and groaned but it did start. I would have bet against it starting but it really did surprise me.

I will be seeing Dr. Fesen on Wednesday at the Heartland Cancer in Great Bend, Kansas. I see Dr. Fesen but I am not scheduled to have any chemo.

Christmas is just about a week away and it looks like it will be a white Christmas this year.

I have an appointment with my family doctor. Dr. Nathan Knackstedt today. He checked my blood pressure. It was 124 over 71 which is really good. Since I don't take any blood pressure meds. He listened to my heart. We then went over my lab reports. He then checked my weight. I have lost 2½ pounds in the last 3 weeks. I will take it you know.

He also changed some of my meds. I was doing 5 mg of Byetta and today he increased it to 10 mg for more complete sugar control. I see Dr. Nathan again in a month, January 17, 2008. Tomorrow I will be seeing Dr. Fesen at the Heartland Center at 9:00 A.M.

December 19, 2007 I made a trip to the cancer center today to keep my appointment with Dr. Fesen, my cancer doctor. He went over my C.T. and bone scans of the past month. He said things were coming along nicely.

He didn't prescribe any new meds or make any changes in my present meds. We set up my schedule for blood tests and chemo for the rest of the year 2007. I have my blood tests the day before Christmas.

My chemo is scheduled on the 26th of December, which is the day after Christmas. A fine finish for 2007. We sometimes wonder why we have all of these terrible diseases. It seems like more and more people, each and every day have developed cancer of some kind.

It seems like many new kinds of cancer are being found in people every day. New drugs and new diets and ways of life are being developed daily. I hope and pray a cure will be found soon.

Christmas weekend. This started with a snowstorm. We had 4 to 6 inches of new snow and a 45 mile an hour wind, making for large snow drifts and very slipper conditions on the roads. We have 12 to 14 inches of snow on the ground. We have had more snow already than we usually get all winter long. Being snowed in is really a bummer. Being at Christmas time makes it even worse.

We have missed church for 3 weeks in a row. Missing church makes for a very long week. It is like having three weeks without any weekends. It has been so bad we have not been able to get out and enjoy the season sights and sounds.

We continue to trust in God. We pray continually, asking Him to take care of us. We still pray even if we don't make it to church. We believe that God will someday take these white spots away. We thank Him daily for all of our many blessings he has bestowed upon us.

Tomorrow is the day before Christmas, or in other words the day of the night before Christmas. I started the day before by going to the Hoisington Hospital or C.B.H. for my blood work. They are to draw the blood tests which include C.B.C., B.M.P. and Mg and P.S.A. So far my P.S.A. continues to be 0.000 and we want to keep it there.

SPECIMEN INQUIRY
HEMATOLOGY

Complete Blood Count

W.B.C.	8.9	4.8-108	k/mm-3
R.B.C.	4.15	4.5-5.9	m/mm-3

Hemoglobin & Hematocrit

Hemoglobin	13.5	13.5-17.5	gm/L
Hematocrit	40.3	40-64	40-64
M.C.V.	97.0	80-100	fl
M.C.H.	32.5	26-34	pd
M.C.H.C.	33.5	32-36	g/dL
R.D.W.	14.8	12-16	%
Platelet Count	248	150-350	k/mm-3
M.P.V.	7.2	7-9	fl
Neutrophils	75.3 H	42-62	%
Lymphocyte	18.2	20-51	%
Monocytes	3.7	1.7-9.3	%

Eosinophil	2.5		0-7	%
Basophil	0.3	H	0.-20	%
Neutrophils #	6.67	H	1.4-6.5	
Lymphocyte #	1.61		1.2-3.4	
Monocyte #	0.33	H	0.1-0.6	
Eosinophil #	0.22		0-0.7	
Basophils #	0.33	H	0.-0.2	k/mm-3

SPECIMEN INQUIRY
CHEMISTRY

Basic Metabolic Profile

Glucose	92		74-106	mg/dL
Bun	14		7-18	mg/dL
Creatinine Serum	0.9	H	0.6-1.3	mg/dL
Bun & Creatinine Ratio	15.00		6.00-2600	
Sodium	140		13.5-155	meg/L
Potassium	3.6		3.5-5.1	meg/L
Chloride	100		98-107	meg/L
Carbon Dioxide	29.7		21-32	mmol
Calcium Level	9.1		8.5-10.1	mg/dL
Osmolality	280		261-280	uosm/k
Magnesium Level	1.7		1.8-2.4	mg/dL

SPECIAL CHEMISTRY

P.S.A. Diagnostic	0.000	0.1-4.1	mg/L
P.S.A. Age Dependent Ranges			

Ages (Years)	40	0.1-1.4
	40-50	0.1-2.0
	50-60	0.1-3.1
	60-70	01-4.1
	70	9.1-4.4

Today is December 26, 2007. I went to the cancer center in Great Bend. My chemo was suppose to be at 9:15 A.M. We were running a little late as we are still battling the weather. We had a lot of snow and wind.

The chemo went very well. My port worked very nicely. I still haven't had any problems with it. The port has been in my chest for nearly 4 years without it plugging up. My Magnesium was very low at 1.6 so they gave me a bag of magnesium through my port. This made my trip longer than I had really planned. I didn't get home until 2:00 P.M.

I will have my last blood test drawn today. The last Monday before New Years day at C.B.H. We don't need an appointment. You just go in and wait your turn. Some mornings you wait just a few minutes and other days you may wait quite a while. One morning I waited for two hours, but what else do I have to do. Today I went right in and no waiting.

Today is Monday. The last day before New Years. Everything is going very well. They hit my vein first stick. My tests were for C.B.C., B.M.P. and Mg. Everything was alright or they would have called me.

They have put me on a maintenance medication as my cancer is under control or in remission, but this doesn't mean everything stops. It just means we now take medication to prevent any future growth. I will continue my blood test and trips to the cancer center every other week for sometime.

I will continue to see Dr. Fesen every 6 weeks for now, at the Heartland Kansas Center. Dr. Fesen had mixed feelings about my chances of recovery in the beginning. I remember him telling me that maybe he could buy me a little time. He will admit this was a miracle.

I came from being paralyzed on one side, unable to get out of bed or go to the restroom on my own, in a wheelchair unable to walk but with Gods help and the hope of a very excellent doctor, Dr. Fesen. I have come back very quickly through prayers from many in the world and the never ending support of my family and church friends.

I have come back to being able to walk and take care of myself. My walking isn't very graceful but I don't care, because I am alive and surviving cancer. My whole outlook on cancer has changed. At one time I was sure cancer was a death certificate. Today I know that cancer run away cell in the body. We all have cells, so we all have the possibility of having cancer.

We need to eat the right foods. Many foods help prevent the growth of cancer cells. We need to pay a lot of attention to our body signals. Our body tells us if something is wrong. We need also, to have regular checkups as regimented by the Medical Community.

Last but not least, by any means is our attitude. We need to keep a very positive feel. We don't set around and mope with a long face and say pity me. We laugh, smile, joke and have a good time. You know it takes more muscles to frown than it does to smile.

Some people may even wonder what you have been, but that is okay. Talk to people all the time. Everyone will feel better if they know they aren't alone in what they are going through. The old saying misery loves company is very true. If you can tell someone else your problems it will make you feel a lot better.

Last but not least, let people know you have cancer. You don't need to hide it. Everyone has health problems of some kind. Get a shirt and wear if proudly. There is nothing about cancer to be ashamed of. Life gave us this problem.

I will talk to anyone who wants to talk about this cancer. Being educated is one thing but we all need to help stamp out cancer. My home is in Hoisington, Kansas. If you want to talk, hunt me up.

I will put a copy of my last lab that was drawn in the back. It was drawn here at Hoisington Hospital C.B.H. Clara Barton Hospital. This lab will contain a C.B.C., B.M.P. and Mg and a P.S.A. complete blood count, basic metabolic profile, magnesium level taken on the last day before New Years 2008.

SPECIMEN INQUIRY
HEMATOLOGY

Complete Blood Count

W.B.C.	9.0		4.8-10.8	k/mm-3
R.B.C.	423	L	4.5-5.9	m/mm-3

Hemoglobin & Hematocrit

Hemoglobin	13.6		13.5-17.5	gm/L
Hematocrit	41.6		50-54	%
M.C.V.	98		80-100	f1
M.C.H.	32.1		26-34	pd
M.C.H.C.	32.7		32-36	g/dL
R.D.W.	15.2		12-16	%
Platelet Count	252		150-350	k/mm-3
M.P.V.	7.3		7-9	f1
Neutrophils	65.6	H	42-62	%
Lymphocyte	23.2		20-51	%
Monocytes	8.8		1.7-9.3	%

Eosinophil	2.1		0-7	%
Basophil	0.3		0-2.0	%
Neutrophils #	5.89		14-6.5	
Lymphocyte #	2.08		1.2-3.4	
Monocyte #	0.79	H	0.1-0.6	
Eosinophil #	0.19		0-0.7	
Basophils #	0.03	H	0-0.2	k/mm-3

SPECIMEN INQUIRY
CHEMISTRY

Comprehensive Metabolic Profile

Glucose	121		74-106	mg/dL
Bun	14		7-18	mg/dL
Creatinine Serum	0.9		0.6-1.3	mg/dL
Bun & Creatinine Ratio	15.00		6.00-2600	
Sodium	143		135-155	meg/L
Potassium	4.0		3.5-5.1	meg/L
Chloride	104		98-107	meg/L
Carbon Dioxide	32.4	H	21-32	mmol/L
Calcium Level	9.2		8.5-10.1	mg/dL
Osmolality	297		261-280	uosm/k9
Albumin/Globulin Ratio	1.6		1.1-2.2	
Bilirubin Total	0.2		02-1.0	mg/dL
AST/SGOT	24		15-37	u/L
Magnesium Level	1.9		1.8-2.4	mg/dL

Alkaline Phosphatase	117	42-128	u/L
ALT-SGPT	50	30-65	u/L

SPECIAL CHEMISTRY

P.S.A. Diagnostic	0.000	0.1-4.1	
Age Dependency Ranges	40	0.1-1.4	ng/nL
	40-50	0.1-2.0	mg/nL
	50-60	0.1-3.1	mg/nL
	60-70	0.1-4.1	mg/nL
	70	0.1-4.4	mg/nL

www.ingramcontent.com/pod-product-compliance
Lightning Source LLC
Chambersburg PA
CBHW031324290526
45784CB00014B/1399